The Architecture of Enough: Hunger, GLP-1, and the Immune Metabolic System

Vyvyane Loh, MD

Published by vlmd Press, 2026.

THE ARCHITECTURE OF ENOUGH: HUNGER, GLP-1, AND THE IMMUNE METABOLIC SYSTEM

First edition. May 10, 2026.

ISBN: 979-8995497912

Written by Vyvyane Loh, MD.

Table of Contents

Praise for *The Architecture of Enough*

"With the precision of a scientist and the grace of a storyteller, Vyvyane Loh reframes the entire conversation around GLP-1. By unifying metabolism and immunity into a single adaptive framework, she reveals why simplistic models fail—and why powerful new therapies demand a more nuanced understanding. Loh illuminates how we evolved for brief, context-dependent GLP-1 signaling, and what changes when those signals become sustained and supraphysiologic. Balanced, insightful, and indispensable for anyone who wants to understand both the promise and the real stakes of these transformative therapies. This is a rare book: scientifically grounded, conceptually fresh, and immediately relevant to modern care. Every physician prescribing these medications, and every patient taking them, should read this."

— **Kenneth M. Ford, PhD**, founder and CEO emeritus of IHMC; founder/co-host of *STEM-Talk.*

"Vyvyane Loh is a brilliant physician-scientist, and a great educator for both providers and patients. This book brings much needed clarity to the mechanisms and stakes of GLP-1 therapy at a time when physicians are being inundated with pressure to prescribe."

— **Guity Valizadeh, MD**, Internal Medicine

A Note to the Reader

This is a book about metabolism, but it is not only a book about metabolism.

It addresses a medication—GLP-1 receptor agonists—because these drugs have changed the way we think about appetite, weight, and metabolic disease. But the real subject of this book is larger. It is about how the body manages energy, how the immune system and metabolism are intertwined, and how modern medicine makes decisions when new therapies arrive faster than understanding.

If you are a patient, you may have encountered GLP-1 medications through your physician, a weight-loss clinic, an online platform, or through friends who are on them. You may be trying to understand how these drugs work and what they mean for your long-term health. If you are a clinician, you may already be prescribing them and grappling with questions that extend beyond guidelines and trial data. Or you might just be a curious reader, interested in how the body regulates hunger, muscle, immunity, and aging, and how these systems hold together under stress.

This book is written for all of you. The most common question I am asked by physicians and patients alike is: *What do you think of these weight loss drugs?* And while the question is the same, I am aware that the concern of each group is nuanced.

Patients want to know:

- Should I be on this drug? What are the side effects?

- Are my health risks from obesity greater than the risks of being on the drug?

- What happens if I stop taking it?

- Will I have to be on it for life?

Physicians want to know:

- Who should I really prescribe this to? If these drugs appear to improve multiple chronic diseases, should more people be on them?

- How do I weigh the risks of long-term therapy against the risks of untreated metabolic disease?

- How do I help patients come off these drugs without significant weight regain?

- If only part of the weight loss is maintained after stopping, what does that mean clinically?

These are questions that cannot be answered meaningfully without a grounding in physiology. GLP-1 medications are often discussed as tools for weight loss. In reality, they sit within a much larger biological system involving the gut, the brain, the immune system, muscle, and the ways the body adapts to changes in energy availability. Understanding that system matters, not only for prescribing medications, but for understanding health itself.

This book runs on two parallel tracks. Each chapter begins with a personal essay. The chapters examine the science of how biological systems regulate energy, and what happens when those systems are overridden. The essays ask a related question: how do we live in a world that no longer knows when to stop? They explore how excess enters every part of our lives, what creates those conditions, and what we mean by enough. These pieces arise from a different kind of inquiry, shaped not only by physiology, but by years of sitting with patients and listening to the ways they live. They ask what kind of world made this science necessary.

In more than two decades of practicing Internal Medicine and Obesity Medicine, I have found that obesity is often misunderstood. It is a disease, and like many chronic diseases, it emerges within the context of how we live. Again and again, I have sat with patients as they described the demands, constraints, and patterns of their lives. What became clear was not a simple chain of individual choices, but a broader mismatch between human biology and the conditions we ask people to endure.

It would be easy to locate the problem in the patient alone, to frame obesity as a failure of discipline, restraint, or will. But that has not been my experience. The pressures, excesses, and absences that shape modern life affect all of us. The essays in this book are written from within that recognition. They are loose social commentaries on the conditions that have shaped our practices in medicine and the problems those conditions have produced. They are informed by what I have observed in myself: the burden of excess, responsibility, and not knowing when to stop. They are also shaped by what I have come to recognize, again and again, in my patients.

It takes time and informed deliberation to understand what is at stake when we use medical interventions to manipulate the body's regulatory systems. This is especially true when the intervention touches hunger, energy, weight, risk, and the long-term architecture of health. While this book begins with a hormone, it ultimately asks a broader question:

How should we think about metabolism, medicine, and the management of energy in the human body, and what happens when we override the systems that tell us when enough is enough?

Chapter 1

Bodies & Battlefields

I first read *The Art of War* as a junior resident.

Internship year was good to me. I had gone to medical school in a city hospital, the best bootcamp for any new recruit, and I arrived at my internship program completely acclimatized to eating dirt, handling scut work while being yelled at, and ready to pull all-nighters with half my brain asleep. Internship at a community hospital was civilized and very bourgie in comparison, and I ended up with a reputation for being competent, careful, and reliable.

July 1st was when we traded our short white coats for the long ones. This was a rite of passage in a highly hierarchical system where the dress code signified your position. Short white coats for medical students and interns, long ones for residents, fellows and Attendings. While there was some measure of flexibility and variance, it was generally accepted and respected. The department had already issued us our long coats and my colleagues had put them on that first day, mostly out of relief that they wouldn't have to launder their grubby, ink-and-coffee stained, now almost light beige short coats. And the crisp, bright whites of the new ones did actually make them look and feel fairly glamorous, motivated and mildly inspired for the first three or four hours, until the daily grind regrounded everyone.

I didn't switch. I tried to, for about 30 minutes, but it felt awkward. My notebooks kept falling out of my pockets when I sat down, the swish of the coat felt limiting as I power-walked to make Grand Rounds on time. Out of irritation, I switched back to my old coat. *It was uncomfortable*, I told my fellow residents and the nurses. But only I knew it wasn't just the coat. It was what it represented.

There is a particular comfort in being the one who executes rather than decides. As an intern, I moved under the guidance of senior residents, fellows, my chief, and Attendings. I could escalate questions, I could defer. As a junior resident, that insulation disappeared. Suddenly, I was leading a team consisting of my new intern, two medical students, and a "Sub-I" or Sub-Intern, a glorified term for a fourth year medical student interning to be an intern (the hierarchy!). While my chief and Attendings were still around for advice and final-tier decisions, I was making the first call on day-to-day clinical decisions. I was responsible not only for my patients, but for the morale, stamina, and coherence of my team.

And even though I had breezed through my internship, medical training still felt like war. Compared to an inner city hospital, my community hospital battlefield was outside the strike zone but still under siege. The language of medicine reinforced it: rounds, 'hits' from the ER, triage, critical care, rapid response, codes. Sleep-deprived teams shuffled from room to room under the eternal day of fluorescent lights, making high-stakes decisions with incomplete information. Now that I was leading my own team, I felt completely inadequate.

I had grown up with the notion that whenever there was a problem, there was also a book with a solution, or at least a guide to dealing with the problem. My approach was to browse my favourite bookstore on a day off, reach mindlessly for a book that 'called' me from a random shelf, and nine out of ten, it would be *The One*. For this imposter syndrome, I adhered to my usual ritual and pulled out a book. *The Art of War*. I stared at the slim volume in my hand. *Wrong book*, I thought, *try again*. But something made me walk to the counter and pay for it instead. Even wrong books can teach you something.

In *The Art of War*, the author, Sun Tzu, warns against battle, a strange stance for a tome on war. He writes that prolonged war exhausts the state. The highest excellence is to win without fighting, and he advises leaders to conserve strength, to understand terrain, to move only when advantage is secured. War, in his framing, is a problem of resource stewardship.That philosophy changed how I ran my team.

I paced our days so no one would burn out. I clarified tasks before rounds so we didn't waste our scarcest resource, time. I doubled down on communication — with nurses, with Attendings, with patients — because miscommunication is friction, and friction wastes energy. I scheduled the day deliberately so we wouldn't be running around in circles, waiting for labs and imaging to be processed. We became known for being swift, efficient and always prepared, and I still got everyone in my team out by 6 pm at the latest.

By the end of residency, I was elected Chief Resident. But the habits that shaped my leadership were forged that first year, under Sun Tzu's quiet discipline. His influence did not remain confined to hospital workflow. It followed me into clinical practice, because medicine, too, is a form of war. Not against patients, but against the medical industrial complex, and the causes of disease: infection, inflammation, metabolic collapse, structural decline. Every intervention is a deployment of force. Every drug is a weapon with a supply chain, collateral effects, and downstream consequences.

Three Philosophies of War

Sun Tzu teaches restraint. Preserve the army; preserve the state; avoid depletion. But he is not the only strategist who has shaped modern thought.

In *On War*, Carl von Clausewitz argues that war is the continuation of politics by other means. If the political objective demands it, escalation is rational. Violence, friction, and loss are not aberrations; they are intrinsic to conflict. Victory may require decisive force.

And then there is Vladimir Lenin, who saw war and crisis not merely as tools of statecraft, but as engines of systemic transformation. Destabilization was not something to avoid; it was something to harness. Collapse could be productive, if it cleared the ground for revolution.

These three philosophies diverge sharply. One prioritizes preservation, another prioritizes political outcome, while the third prioritizes structural overthrow. Medicine today, particularly in the era of pharmaceutical dominance, often resembles Clausewitz — and at times, Lenin — more than Sun Tzu.

We escalate quickly and target endpoints aggressively, accepting side effects as the cost of achieving metric-defined victory. We think nothing of destabilizing physiology in order to reconstruct it. Sometimes that may be necessary, but sometimes, in our pursuit of endpoints, we exhaust the very system we are trying to preserve.

Beyond the practice of medicine, I've come to realize that the body is a battlefield. Our immune system stands ready to defend us from toxins and enemy microbes. But every army needs resources, fuel, supplies. Sun Tzu's framework mirrors metabolic regulation, avoidance of inflammatory overdrive, management of immune activation without collapse, and expansion/growth that does not destroy the body.

Metabolism is not a static target. It is an adaptive system, with immune tone as its regulatory force. Appetite, inflammation, muscle, bone, and brain are not isolated battlefields but interdependent terrains. The question is not whether we fight disease but how.

We start, not with a drug, but with a relationship.

Before GLP-1 became a medication, before obesity became a diagnosis category, before metabolism was reduced to calories burned and calories stored, was the body's ancient language of fuel, defense, repair, and identity. Metabolism does not simply power the immune system like gasoline in an engine. It helps determine what immune cells become, how they behave, what they remember, and what they are prepared to defend.

To understand GLP-1, then, we have to begin upstream. We have to begin with the immune-metabolic system itself: the living architecture through which the body decides what is threat, what is nourishment, what is repair, and what is enough.

In the Beginning

The first life forms separated themselves from the environment with a boundary, a membrane that allowed for selectivity as to what to keep out and what to hold in. But a boundary alone was not enough. To survive, a cell also needed a way to capture energy and a way to use it to maintain itself. From the beginning, life required an Energy and Resource Management Department. We now call it Metabolism.

Metabolism has two major divisions. The anabolic division builds. It constructs the physical structures that allow the cell to function, such as DNA, proteins, membranes, and receptors. The catabolic division is for demolition. It breaks down and dismantles chemical compounds, releasing energy stored within them. Some of the pieces can be recycled as raw materials, chemical skeletons that can be used to build new structures. So at its core, metabolism is the extraction of energy from internal and external resources and the use of that energy and those materials to sustain life.

The energy currency of the cell is a molecule called ATP or adenosine triphosphate. As its name suggests, it contains three phosphate groups linked together. When the cell needs energy, one of these phosphate groups is removed in a chemical reaction called hydrolysis. This reaction releases usable energy that powers cellular work, from muscle contraction to DNA replication to immune activation.

Metabolism is maintained by complex biochemical reactions and enzymes. Overseeing this chemistry are hormones related to how we make and use energy. Just like insulin, glucagon and cortisol, GLP-1 is a hormone made by certain tissues and sent through the blood to the body to affect your metabolism.

Energy Sensing: How the Cell Decides

Our cells do not build, burn, store, or mobilize energy at random. Before we do anything, our bodies need to know the cost. What resources do we have, how much can we spend? To do this, our cells continuously measure their internal environment and adjust accordingly. Two major molecular systems act as energy sensors and help the cell make these decisions: **AMPK** and **mTOR.**

These act as energy gauges that feed into systems to help us conserve and restore energy, or allow us to spend it on building projects and other needs. When AMPK is activated, it means that ATP is being used up. This tells the cell that it is running short on fuel and should switch to conservation measures. mTOR registers when we have abundant nutrients and fuel in the form of glucose, amino acids, cholesterol. It also responds to growth signals and other signs that the cell is running on a full tank. These two sensors work together to give a running tab of the energy status in the cell: when energy is plentiful, mTOR rises, AMPK falls, and the system is allowed to build.

This balance allows cells to adapt to feast and famine, growth and stress, infection and recovery. *Adaptation* is the key word here. The word metabolism comes from the Greek *metabolē*, meaning 'change'. A robust metabolism detects, handles, and channels energy flux within the cell. Just like an army, a cell must be able to **shift its energy strategies** depending on internal and external conditions in order to survive. One that cannot adjust to changing circumstances will not last.

What About Oxygen?

In order to burn food for energy, we need oxygen. So it makes sense for the cell to have an oxygen sensor as well. HIF-1α is a protein that becomes active when oxygen levels fall or when cells experience inflammatory stress. This sends a signal to re-wire metabolism to support the inflamed cell and help it survive.

In obesity, fat cells often swell to store more energy, but the body cannot make blood vessels quickly enough to keep up with the enlarging fat cells. Just like adding five bathrooms at once to your home without increasing water and sewage lines, less blood is able to flow through the fat cells. There is less oxygen available per cell resulting in mild, chronic inflammation, and HIF-1α is activated. It turns on genes that instruct the cell to send out signaling molecules called cytokines. The Mayday they send reads: *help, our energy supply is falling!* And in response, the body diverts its energy and resources to the failing cells.

The bottom line is that your metabolism is a sophisticated system to generate, manage and allocate energy to your body. All living things need energy. Stop your metabolism and you're dead.

The Energy Cost of Inflammation

Your immune system is your Department of Defence and inflammation is a process whereby the body summons its military to protect and defend against damage done to it. And like any functioning militia, it requires a budget to maintain, and a different one to deploy the troops.

When your immune soldiers are activated, there is an energy cost. Even mild chronic inflammation seen in rheumatoid arthritis or obesity can increase resting energy expenditure by 5–15%. Assuming energy consumption to be 2000 kcal/day, this would approximate to 100-300 kcal more per day, depending on age, sex, body composition and other factors.

The energy is spent on prepping for battle. We enlarge the troops by making more immune cells. Increasing blood pressure and heart rate pumps more blood to the body as the circulation is the supply line to the battle front. We engage the Signal Corps for communication by making signaling molecules (cytokines) and acute-phase reactants. Think of these as war sirens to alert the body to danger. And finally, we need to build, make and repair structures, energy and other resources (substrate cycling).

Fever increases energy demand even further. For each 1°C (~1.8°F) rise in body temperature, metabolic rate increases by approximately 10–13%. A 2°C (~3.6°F) fever may increase energy expenditure by 20% or more. In severe inflammation such as sepsis, major burns, or critical illness, metabolic rate can increase dramatically, sometimes by 30–60% above baseline. In these settings, the body often becomes profoundly catabolic, breaking down muscle and fat to sustain the immune response.

Energy Reallocation During Inflammation

But the body doesn't just burn more calories with inflammation. It reallocates fuel as several coordinated changes occur. Peripheral insulin resistance develops. Normally, insulin helps the body move excess glucose into fat, muscle and the liver. The glucose is stored as glycogen in muscle and liver, and in fat cells, it is stored as a fat called triacyl-glycerol or triglyceride. With insulin resistance, tissues become less sensitive to insulin action.

With a lessened ability to move into fat, muscle and liver, the glucose remains in the bloodstream, readily available to fuel immune cells. Another normal function of insulin is to prevent fatty acids from leaving the fat cell. These fatty acids are usually bound three at a time to a glucose-derived molecule called glycerol. When that happens we form a molecule of triacyl-glycerol. That is why you commonly hear that "insulin makes fat", a process called lipogenesis. It does so to prevent high levels of glucose in the blood which can damage organs.

With insulin resistance, insulin's actions are not as effective despite having more insulin on board. This means it is less able to keep the triacyl-glycerols from breaking up back into glycerol and fatty acids (lipolysis) which leak out of the fat cell. Free fatty acids are very toxic and cause a lot of damage to the body. However, in this context they provide more energy to immune cells and damaged (inflamed) tissue.

Additionally, breakdown of protein and muscle occurs. The amino acids resulting from this breakdown and lipolysis (fat breakdown) provide the liver with substrates to make more glucose (gluconeogenesis). We also use some of these substrates to make acute-phase proteins (the sirens) and carrier vehicles called VLDL to transport fats for fuel to different parts of the body.

These shifts are not random and prioritize certain tissues over others. So who receives the fuel?

- Immune cells, which rely heavily on glucose and often use insulin-independent transport.

- The liver, which produces acute-phase proteins such as C-reactive protein, fibrinogen, complement proteins, and hepcidin.

- The brain, which mediates sickness behavior — fatigue, reduced appetite, social withdrawal — adaptive responses that conserve energy and limit spread of infection.

So inflammation isn't simply heat and swelling but a coordinated metabolic redirection of energy resources to the immune system.

An immune response is not a simple switch that goes on or off. Instead, as inflammatory signals increase, the body shifts through distinct metabolic states. In mild activation, immune cells temporarily increase glucose use to respond quickly. The metabolic shift is short-lived and usually resolves once the threat passes. With moderate inflammation, the body begins reallocating fuel: skeletal muscle reduces glucose uptake; adipose tissue reduces storage; the liver increases glucose production. These changes ensure that glucose is available to immune cells and the liver.

In severe inflammation, metabolic rate rises substantially. Just as household and community items were recycled in WWII to make weapons, the body breaks down muscle and fat to sustain immune activity and acute-phase protein production. Energy production becomes less efficient as mitochondria (the energy factories in cells) experience stress, and muscle mass declines. At this level, metabolism is no longer balanced between building and breakdown, and catabolism dominates. If prolonged, this state can lead to cachexia, a state of accelerated and advanced muscle loss.

Metabolic Switches Shape Immune Function

Earlier, we described how cells sense energy availability through systems such as AMPK, mTOR, and HIF-1α. These systems monitor fuel, nutrients, and environmental stress. They not only regulate metabolism but also help determine how immune cells behave.

Besides energy, an immune response also requires instruction as immune cells must decide whether to expand, restrain, or escalate. Metabolic signals provide part of that instruction.

mTOR: Permission to Build

When nutrients are abundant and energy is sufficient, mTOR activity rises. In immune cells, this supports troop expansion and production of protein structures to support inflammation.

An activated immune system must build. It must produce cytokines, antibodies, receptors, and new cells. These are construction projects, and mTOR provides the signal that resources are available. With mTOR active, immune responses can expand and progress.

AMPK: The Brake and the Checkpoint

When cellular energy falls, AMPK activity increases. In immune cells, this shift favors energy conservation, reduced building and production, and more restraint in battle.

Inflammation is costly. It cannot continue indefinitely without consequence. AMPK helps ensure that immune activation does not outpace available resources. This is where Sun Tzu's advice becomes life-saving: *Preserve the army; preserve the state; avoid depletion.* If mTOR permits building, AMPK asks whether the system can afford it. Together, they create balance between expansion and restraint.

HIF-1α: The Signal of Urgency

When oxygen delivery is limited or when inflammatory stress alters the cellular environment, HIF-1α turns on genes to produce energy quickly though less efficiently. This is because when the cell is under siege, speed matters more than efficiency. HIF-1α supports rapid response under stress to generate energy.

Metabolism as Instruction

These metabolic switches do more than supply fuel because they also influence immune identity.

Cells in a growth-permissive state behave differently from cells in a conservation state. Those operating under the stress of oxygen deprivation behave differently from those in stable conditions. Metabolism helps determine whether the immune system escalates, restrains, or resolves.

IL-6: A Messenger Between Systems

Among the molecules that link metabolism and immunity, IL-6 is a cytokine (signaling molecule) that plays a distinctive and complex role.

IL-6 is released by immune cells during inflammation. It is also released by skeletal muscle during exercise. It mobilizes glucose, signals the liver to produce acute-phase proteins, and alters substrate use across tissues. IL-6 moves at the intersection between the immune system and metabolism.

In this way, IL-6 illustrates a broader principle: the immune system and metabolic system are not separate networks but are intertwined. When metabolic signaling shifts, immune behavior shifts with it, and energy management becomes immune instruction.

Obesity and Its Effects on Metabolism

Contrary to what people believe, obesity doesn't happen because of a 'slow metabolism'. In fact, people with obesity have a higher resting metabolic rate, meaning their energy expenditure per hour is higher than someone without obesity. Part of it is due to the body's compensatory mechanisms to use more energy, body mass/fat-free mass mass and total body tissue load, and also the energy costs of chronic mild to moderate inflammation that occurs with obesity.

In obesity, there is a net positive energy gain between what you take in and how much you spend. This cannot simply be accounted for by an equation because your metabolism has intricate sensors and diversions to sense and re-direct energy. You can think of it as akin to money-laundering.

In this situation, money that was gained illegally is re-directed in the financial system through elaborate schemes. These involve setting up legitimate businesses to mix both legal and illegal sources of income, re-directing money through diverse cash and electronic purchases, and eventually re-investing the money into legitimate businesses. In this way, money-laundering drains the economy of trillions of dollars. Tracing the flow of illegally earned money is very costly and yields very little success.

So while it may seem simple enough to calculate your energy difference by subtracting energy spent from your energy intake, the math (which is usually an approximation at best) does not always add up.

Bottom Line

Metabolism is about sensing and allocation of resources.

Like money-laudering, it is not easy to trace energy flow in and out of the body.

So far, we've looked at three core environmental sensors:

- AMPK → Is there enough energy?
- mTOR → Are there enough nutrients to build?
- HIF-1α → Is the environment stressed or oxygen-limited?

Together they answer:

- Can we build?
- Should we conserve?
- Are we under threat?

Once a cell or organism answers these questions, it must decide where energy goes. Energy can be:

- Produced (ATP generation)
- Stored (glycogen, fat)
- Mobilized (lipolysis, proteolysis)
- Redirected (gluconeogenesis, acute-phase protein synthesis)
- Signaled across tissues (insulin, glucagon, IL-6)

Inflammation increases demand. As immune activation escalates from mild to severe, metabolic cost rises and fuel is reallocated. Metabolic signals influence whether immune cells expand, restrain, or escalate.

The immune system is metabolically powered, and metabolic systems are shaped by immune signals. They are interdependent networks responding to changing constraints. Thus, **when manipulating metabolism, we are never only manipulating weight**.

****

Chapter 2

Around 860AD, Chinese scholar Duan Chengshi collected his notes on his travels and personal observations of nature and popular culture. That 30-volume text became the *Miscellanies of You-yang*. In it he described a flat, chisel-headed creature that preyed on earthworms by encircling them and dissolving their bodies with a neurotoxin. He wrote that it could separate into pieces, highlighting its unique ability to multiply and regenerate. We now think he might have been describing the Hammerhead worm, a land planarian so toxic that chickens died from pecking it.

Planaria are mushy flatworms with triangular heads that bear two eyespots. They are the original hydra as their stem cells allow them to regenerate all organs and tissue. A gecko that loses its tail can grow a new one, but its tail cannot grow the rest of the body. It is discarded, useless after its amputation. If you cut a planarian in half, each piece becomes a full-fledged planarian. Cut it into three parts and you end up with three planarians. The record so far has been to generate 279 individual planarians from cutting one into 279 pieces. Every single fragment is biologically viable.

What is remarkable about this is that they must decide what to become. When severed, the fragment that was once tail must recognize that it is no longer whole, no longer *enough* to survive. It must know that a head is missing. And the fragment that once bore eyes must register the absence of a tail. Polarity must be re-established, axes redrawn to reorganize chaos into patterns. They do this with an internal GPS regulated by Positional Control Genes (PCGs) to constantly map the body so that any damage can be located within its inner topography and new parts regenerated from stem cells.

In 2015, a batch of *Dugesia japonica* planarians spent five weeks in space. Before they were loaded onto SpaceX CRS-5, fifteen worms had their heads and tails snipped off and placed along with ten intact worms into a sealed tube filled half with air and half with spring water. Once they were on board the International Space Station they were subjected to experiments to see how microgravity and space radiation affected their physiology.

The most spectacular result from these studies was the emergence of the Janus Worm. Under the near-zero gravity conditions in the space station, one headless and tailless worm regenerated not one, but two heads. This had never happened in over 18 years of experiments with these animals.

But it was when the worms were returned to earth that scientists realized the extent of change that they had undergone. Immediately after landing they curled up as if stunned by their re-entry and only regained their mobility after two hours. Even twenty months later they were different. They were less photophobic than ordinary worms, as if the darkness of space had made them crave light. Their metabolism changed, along with their microbiome. They were more unpredictable, more apt to split into two spontaneously, dividing in fission like unstable atoms. The Janus worm continued to regenerate two heads when both ends were decapitated. From generation to generation this double-headed form persisted. What interested me most was not simply that the worm had changed, but that the change endured after return.

I often think about the worms when I think of home. I left Singapore when I was a teenager, first for boarding school, and then for college. At first I was terribly homesick and missed everything but of course, life continues in your absence. Roads change, buildings arise and disappear, and trees are sacrificed for highways. Since then I've always returned as a familiar stranger. Suddenly you are no longer inside the jokes. There are new Singlish words I don't understand. *You can't go home again*, Thomas Wolfe wrote, not as the same person anyway.

We leave for the stars only to discover they are rocks, and the space we craved is cold and lacks gravity. It shapes us, thinning sinew and bone, sapping strength until we are as emptied out as it is. And then upon return, shriveled, crushed by the heaviness of air, vertigo-sick from gravity, we look sunwards, taking the light in greedily with our two heads.

To understand what GLP-1 drugs do, we first have to understand the biological family they borrow from.

The body's own GLP-1 system is brief, local, and highly contextual. Pharmacologic GLP-1 receptor agonists are longer-acting, more sustained, and more forceful. They do not simply "replace" the body's GLP-1. They extend, amplify, and redirect parts of a signaling system that was never designed to act as a single isolated lever.

This chapter begins with that system: where GLP-1 comes from, how its family members behave, how the GLP-1 drugs were discovered, and the difference between a physiological signal and a pharmacologic one.

The Mother Molecule

Every biological system has its matriarch, the one molecule from which all the others descend. For metabolism, that figure is proglucagon, the Mother Molecule.

From this single, unassuming precursor, a whole lineage of hormones is born: **glucagon, glicentin, GLP-1, GLP-2, oxyntomodulin**, and others still being defined. Each carries a different temperament, a different message, and often, a different tissue of origin. And yet, all trace their ancestry to the same gene.

The Accidental Hormone (1920s)

John Raymond Murlin and Charles P. Kimball were researchers working in the early 1920s, just after insulin had been isolated. At the time, insulin was extracted from pancreatic tissue to treat diabetes, but something odd kept happening: When crude pancreatic extracts were injected into animals, blood glucose sometimes **rose** instead of falling.

That was unexpected because everyone knew, of course, that insulin lowers glucose. So Murlin and Kimball separated the pancreatic extracts into fractions. One fraction was insulin which lowered glucose. Another fraction raised glucose. In 1923, they published evidence of a "hyperglycemic substance" from the pancreas and named it **glucagon**, literally: *glucose + agonist* (a substance that drives glucose up)

They knew very little about this substance, not its sequence, not its receptor or its role aside from countering insulin to raise blood sugar. Glucagon was recognized primarily as insulin's opposite.

The Long Silence (1930s–1960s)

For decades, glucagon lived in insulin's shadow as its antagonist. Insulin was made in the beta-cells of the pancreas. Glucagon, on the other hand, was found to be a pancreatic alpha-cell hormone that stimulates the liver to make glucose, thereby opposing insulin and raising blood sugar during fasting.

However, its molecular identity remained unclear. In the 1950s and 60s, improved purification methods allowed scientists to isolate glucagon more precisely. Eventually its amino acid sequence was determined as a 29-amino-acid peptide.

Still, something strange lingered. When scientists examined pancreatic tissue and intestinal tissue, they noticed immunoreactive material that looked like glucagon but wasn't exactly glucagon. There were ***glucagon-like*** peptides that no one yet understood.

The Molecular Era (1970s–1980s)

The turning point came with molecular biology. Researchers cloned the gene responsible for glucagon production. What they discovered was astonishing: there was no "glucagon gene." Instead, there was a **larger precursor gene** encoding a big protein that contained glucagon embedded within it. This precursor was named **proglucagon**.

It turns out that proglucagon wasn't just glucagon with a tail that could be lopped off to create the active hormone. It contained within it glucagon, GLP-1 (glucagon-like peptide-1), GLP-2, oxyntomodulin, and glicentin. All in one sequence. But the real revelation? It turned out that **different tissues processed the same precursor differently.**

In pancreatic alpha cells: The enzyme PCSK2 cuts proglucagon→Result: glucagon is released.

In intestinal L-cells: The enzyme PCSK1/3 cuts it differently→Result: GLP-1, GLP-2, oxyntomodulin are formed.

Same gene, same Mother Molecule cut by different scissors. That discovery reframed everything. Glucagon was not a solitary hormone but just one cleavage product of a multi-hormone precursor. And GLP-1, hidden inside the same Mother Molecule all this while, was not a separate evolutionary innovation.

Proglucagon can be functionally thought of as a manuscript. And like any manuscript, it depends on the editor. In pancreatic alpha cells, one set of enzymes shapes it one way. In intestinal L-cells, another editor (enzyme) arrives, and the story changes. As any writer knows, it's all in the edits.

The Incretin Twist (1980s–1990s)

Once GLP-1 was isolated from intestinal extracts, researchers discovered its *incretin effect*, that is, it stimulated insulin secretion in a glucose-dependent manner (see box). But unlike insulin or glucagon, GLP-1 was rapidly degraded by an enzyme called DPP-4 and had a very short half-life of barely 2 ½ minutes.

Only about 10% of the secreted hormone reaches the bloodstream. This is not an error of biology but a sophisticated, coordinated system based on the family of proglucagon products and other gut hormones. Hunger and restraint, mobilization and storage, stress and restoration–these are the fluctuating conditions in life and the system was never designed for permanent satiety or permanent suppression. Instead it is a family of hormones juggling alternating signals that respond to need in order to achieve homeostatic balance.

The Incretin Effect

Jean La Barre introduced the term *incretin* in the 1930s. But the concept traces back even earlier.

In 1902, William Bayliss and Ernest Starling discovered **secretin**, the first hormone, which stimulated pancreatic bicarbonate secretion. That discovery introduced the concept of "**hormones**" — internal chemical messengers.

Soon after, scientists began wondering: if the gut releases a hormone to stimulate pancreatic exocrine secretion (*exocrine*: substances secreted into ducts that lead to cavities such as your intestines), does it release something that stimulates pancreatic **endocrine** secretion (*endocrine*: substances secreted directly into the bloodstream) also — in this case, insulin?

By the 1920s–30s, experiments showed that oral glucose triggered a stronger insulin response than intravenous glucose. This implied that something from the gut enhanced insulin secretion. La Barre proposed that this hypothetical gut hormone should be called an **incretin,** a substance that stimulates insulin.

It was a functional name, not a molecular one. The molecule was yet unknown...

Glucagon: The Ancient Signal

Glucagon was the first family member of the proglucagon family to be discovered and entered the scientific stage in 1923 as insulin's antagonist — a hyperglycemic extract from the pancreas identified by John Raymond Murlin and Charles P. Kimball. Naming GLP-1 (glucagon-like peptide-1) after glucagon is like tagging *Junior* to a name to signify someone's offspring. To learn about the child we must first understand its parent, and its origin story.

For decades, glucagon's identity seemed straightforward: A 29–amino acid peptide

released from pancreatic alpha-cells to stimulate liver glucose production during fasting. In short, insulin stored fuel (anabolic) while glucagon mobilized it (catabolic).

The Assay Problem

In the 1950s and 60s, hormone measurement entered a new era with the development of radioimmunoassay (RIA), pioneered by Rosalyn Yalow and colleagues. RIA transformed endocrinology. For the first time, tiny hormone concentrations could be measured in blood.

But early glucagon assays had a flaw in that they were not specific. The antibodies used in those early assays often recognized **multiple proglucagon-derived peptides**, not just pancreatic glucagon. This is because scientists at that time did not yet fully understand that along with glucagon came a slew of family members.

Early assays frequently detected glucagon, oxyntomodulin, glicentin, and "enteroglucagon" (a term used in the 1960s–70s for gut-derived glucagon-like material). They were measuring "glucagon-immunoreactivity" and not pure pancreatic glucagon.

Finally, from the 1990s to 2000s, more specific assays were developed. These two-site sandwich assays targeted the exact 29 amino acid sequence, leading to a clearer distinction between pancreatic glucagon and other fragments. Only then did we begin to understand what glucagon levels actually were in health and disease, and the significance of the proglucagon family in metabolic regulation.

What This Meant

For years, glucagon was blamed for metabolic dysfunction in ways that were not always precise. If "glucagon" appeared elevated in type 2 diabetes, was it true pancreatic glucagon or cross-reactive intestinal peptides that contaminated the assays? If glucagon seemed present in unexpected contexts, was that physiology, or assay artifact?

As assays improved, glucagon revealed something more nuanced. As the big sister of the proglucagon family, its significance is seen in its multiple roles:

- It is essential for amino acid clearance.

- It regulates nitrogen disposal in the liver.

- It protects against hypoglycemia.

- It coordinates fasting metabolism.

It is not simply a glucose-raising nuisance but a survival hormone.

The Liver–Alpha Cell Axis

The last two decades have revealed an unexpected discovery. It turns out that glucagon secretion is tightly linked to circulating amino acids. When amino acids rise, pancreatic alpha cells release glucagon which signals the liver to make glucose (gluconeogenesis), produce an excretion product called urea (ureagenesis), and in doing so, clear amino acids from the blood.

If liver glucagon signaling is impaired, amino acids accumulate. Alpha cells respond by proliferating and secreting more glucagon. This feedback loop is now called the **liver–alpha cell axis**.

This axis reframes glucagon not just as a counterweight to insulin, but as a regulator of protein economy; not just a glucose hormone, but a nitrogen steward.

The Conversation Between Pancreas and Liver

Imagine eating a protein-rich meal–steak, fish, eggs. Once absorbed, amino acids (the building blocks of protein) rise in the bloodstream. These are used to make hormones, cellular structures, receptors, muscle cells. Any excess that is not used by the body is passed out in urine.

Amino acids are so named because they carry a nitrogen group in their structure, called an amino group ($-NH_2$). Protein metabolism results in the formation of ammonia (NH_3) which is toxic to the body. The ammonia is brought to the liver where it is converted to an inert substance called urea which can then be removed in the urine. What we've only recently discovered in the last decade is glucagon's role in this process.

Today we recognize that:

- Amino acids stimulate glucagon secretion.

- Glucagon prompts the uptake of amino acid <uptake> into the liver for detoxification by removing the amino group and forming urea which is removed in the urine.

- Impaired glucagon signaling in the liver blocks this process and leads to high amino acid levels in the blood (hyperaminoacidemia).

- Hyperaminoacidemia signals the need for more glucagon and drives the growth of alpha-cells in the pancreas to produce high glucagon levels.

It became clear that glucagon is not merely opposing insulin but also **maintaining amino acid homeostasis by coordinating protein metabolism with glucose production**. This keeps nitrogen from becoming toxic in the form of ammonia.

This feedback loop, the liver–alpha cell axis, has even prompted calls by researchers for a name change. Instead of glucagon (*glucose* + *agonist*, meaning glucose producing), perhaps it should be called *proteinon*, or *aminoacidon*. While unlikely to happen, it should highlight the hormone's role in protein metabolism.

In numerous experiments with glucagon deficiency models (glucagon knock-out mice or those with genetic alpha-cell deletions), the animals continued to make glucose in their liver and did not die from low blood sugar (hypoglycemia). Instead, profound defects were seen in the liver's detoxification of amino acids, resulting in drastic impairment of its ability to convert them to urea. It turns out that glucagon's essential role is to regulate protein metabolism and that its role in glucose production is largely secondary. Sadly, despite its critical implications to our understanding of physiology, this two decades old scientific discovery is still not taught in the medical curriculum today.

When the Liver Loses Responsiveness

Now back to our protein-rich meal which has been digested and the amino acids absorbed into the blood. What happens if glucagon's signal to the liver is muted as can occur in hepatic insulin resistance and fatty liver disease? (In experimental studies it has been achieved through glucagon receptor blockade or genetic disruption of glucagon signaling.)

The alpha cells still sense rising amino acids and release glucagon, but the liver is unable to respond fully. Amino acids remain elevated and the pancreatic alpha-cells interpret this as insufficient signaling or a deficiency in glucagon, and release more glucagon in response.

Consider a patient with metabolic dysfunction and fatty liver. After meal amino acids remain elevated longer than expected, and glucagon levels are chronically higher than in lean controls. For years, we erroneously believed that it is this elevated glucagon level that has a key role in causing high blood sugar. We termed it *glucagon excess* without realizing that it is actually an adaptive response,

Under chronic muting of the glucagon signal (even as extra glucagon is being secreted), the alpha-cells proliferate, forming more alpha-cells in an attempt to compensate for this glucagon resistance. This *alpha-cell hyperplasia* or expansion of alpha-cell tissue is the pancreas' way of responding adaptively to disrupted amino acid balance in the body.

The Many Offspring of Proglucagon

When glucagon was first purified in the mid-20th century, it appeared self-contained: a 29–amino acid peptide with a clear job to raise glucose. But in the 1980s, molecular cloning unsettled that simplicity. Researchers isolated the gene that encoded glucagon, expecting to find a short blueprint. Instead they found a long molecule with a molecular weight that was five to six times larger than a mature glucagon molecule. What were all these extra "bits" in proglucagon?

As it turns out, the Mother Molecule had embedded within it multiple peptides (protein chains) arranged in sequence, waiting to be cut. This redefined our understanding of glucagon as not just a lone signal but one fragment of a larger design.

One Manuscript, Different Editors

The cleavage of proglucagon depends on location. The difference lies in the enzymes known as prohormone convertases. One type is predominant in the pancreas while another is active in the intestine. In the intestine, L-cells express a set of enzymes called PCSK 1 and 3 which cut proglucagon to yield GLP-1, GLP-2, oxyntomodulin, and glicentin. These same enzymes process proglucagon in the brain.

In the pancreas, alpha-cells express PCSK 2, which cuts proglucagon primarily into glucagon, glycentin-related polypeptide (GRPP), intervening peptide-1 (IP-1), and major proglucagon fragment (MPGF).

However, under **metabolic stress, islet inflammation, or when insulin-making beta-cells are damaged, pancreatic alpha-cells can shift their processing to include PCSK 1/3, producing GLP-1**. Thus, these cells have been found to "moonlight" as producers of bioactive GLP-1 to aid in glucose control in the pancreas when needed.

The GLP-1 produced by the alpha-cells now act to **inhibit glucagon secretion**, directly and through indirect pathways. Interestingly, the effect of GLP-1 on glucagon is glucose-dependent. While it inhibits glucagon during high or normal glucose levels (as seen in the fed state), research in mouse models suggests it may actually help stimulate glucagon during hypoglycemia, acting as a protective "safety switch" to prevent dangerously low blood sugar.

Primary vs. Extra-Intestinal Sources of GLP-1

Site	Enzyme profile	Key physiological role
Distal ileal & colonic L-cells	PC1/3 → GLP-1, GLP-2, oxyntomodulin	Nutrient-triggered incretin and "ileal brake" signaling via vagal afferents
Nucleus tractus solitarius (NTS) neurons in the caudal brainstem	PC1/3	Central GLP-1 that projects to hypothalamus, amygdala, parabrachial nucleus, VTA, etc.—controls appetite, stress, cardiovascular tone
Pancreatic α-cells under metabolic stress or β-cell failure	PC1/3 up-regulation in some α-cells → local GLP-1	Paracrine protection of β-cells and local insulin–glucagon coordination
Lung and heart	Low-level transcripts	Paracrine/repair roles post-injury; animal data

Enter GIP

GLP-1 does not act alone in the incretin response. GIP (glucose-dependent insulinotropic polypeptide) is secreted from K-cells in the part of the intestine that is closer to the stomach (the proximal intestine). It is the product of the GIP gene. While not descended from proglucagon (we could perhaps think of it as an in-law), it too, amplifies insulin secretion after meals.

After a meal, GIP levels rise first in the proximal gut, followed by GLP-1 further away in the distal gut. In this way they are co-activated, temporally staggered, spatially segregated and often physiologically antagonistic. This staggered release is not accidental and reflects **phased nutrient handling**:

- **GIP** → early storage signal (tells body to extract and store nutrients)

- **GLP-1** → downstream braking, signal to stop eating towards the end of the meal

It should be noted that GIP behaves differently in metabolic disease. In type 2 diabetes (DM2), GIP's insulin stimulating effect diminishes while GLP-1's effect does not. The two hormones give off parallel signals that provide redundancy and nuance.

Coordination and Feedback

The members of the proglucagon family do not merely act outward. They also feed back into the system.

GLP-1 suppresses glucagon secretion acutely. Glucagon influences hepatic amino acid metabolism, which in turn influences alpha-cell signaling. Oxyntomodulin has complex dual effects, interacting with glucagon and GLP-1 receptors. GLP-2 alters nutrient absorption, changing the metabolic substrate delivered to the liver.

In nature, no peptide acts in isolation. Each adjusts the tone of the others. This should be regarded as a family of hormones, involved in the 'family business' of metabolism, and not a solo act.

The Rhythm of Release

Physiologically, this family operates in pulses: meal arrives, the L-cells (intestine) and alpha-cells (pancreas) respond, signals peak. Enzymes degrade them quickly so that the half-life of native GLP-1 is measured in minutes.

Short-lived signals prevent dominance by allowing flexibility and oscillation. Proglucagon products rise and fall like notes in a musical score. When one swells, others recede. The system works in rhythmic synchrony as a coordinated orchestra.

A Family, Not Fragments

Remember the planarians? Cutting one produces two planarian fragments that are each biologically viable. They each regenerate and become complete, living planarians. Proglucagon doesn't produce isolated hormones that act independently. Each time it is cut, there are **equal ratios of its products**. In the intestines, proglucagon cleavage doesn't just give us GLP-1 but **1:1 ratios** of GLP-1, GLP-2, glicentin/oxyntomodulin.

Each has a slightly different role.

- GLP-1 enhances insulin secretion and slows gastric emptying.

- GLP-2 supports intestinal growth and barrier integrity.

- Oxyntomodulin can bind both glucagon and GLP-1 receptors, subtly modulating energy expenditure and intake.

- Glicentin modulates gastric acid, motility; has possible growth effects on the gut.

They are released **together** to coordinate nutrient absorption, blood sugar control, satiety, and intestinal adaptation.

Hormone / Peptide	Primary Source	Main Physiologic Action	Role in Metabolic Balance
Glucagon	Pancreatic α-cells	↑ Hepatic glucose output; ↑ amino acid uptake; ↑ lipolysis	Maintains fuel and amino acid supply during fasting, illness, stress
GLP-1	Intestinal L-cells; brainstem (NTS)	↑ Glucose dependent insulin; ↓ glucagon; slows gastric emptying; ↑ satiety	Coordinates nutrient inflow with insulin, appetite, and immune tone
GLP-2	Intestinal L-cells	Promotes mucosal growth, repair, and barrier integrity	Preserves gut structure, absorption, and limits immune activation from barrier failure
Oxyntomodulin	Intestinal L-cells	Weak GLP-1R + glucagon receptor agonist; ↓ food intake; ↑ energy expenditure	Integrates satiety with energy use; natural "dual-signal" on GLP-1/ glucagon axis
Glicentin	Intestinal L-cells	Modulates gastric acid, motility; possible trophic gut effects	Coordinates digestive timing and luminal environment, indirectly supporting nutrient handling
MPGF (Major Proglucagon Fragment)	Pancreatic α-cells	Processing intermediate; unclear direct endocrine role	Reflects tissue-specific processing rather than a key systemic hormone (placeholder in the family)

GLP-1 Beyond the Gut

For years, GLP-1 was thought to be purely intestinal and termed a 'gut hormone'. But we now know that proglucagon is also made in neurons in the brainstem, particularly in an area called the nucleus tractus solitarius (NTS). There, GLP-1 is produced centrally in response to neural and visceral inputs.

GLP-1 signaling, therefore, exists in three domains:

- Intestinal (nutrient-triggered release)

- Pancreatic (local modulation within islets)

- Central (brainstem production influencing appetite and autonomic tone)

Thus it is important to note that the molecule travels via the blood (endocrine action), and also acts locally (paracrine action) within the gut and in the brain.

GLP-1 in the Brain — The Central Circuit

GLP-1 is also a neuropeptide, with prominent effects in the brain. Proglucagon is made in a specific population of neurons located primarily in the nucleus tractus solitarius (NTS) in the brainstem which sits on top of the spinal cord. These neurons synthesize proglucagon and process it into GLP-1. Unlike intestinal GLP-1, which is rapidly degraded before it enters the circulation, central GLP-1 acts locally, within neural circuits.

The NTS is not an arbitrary location as it is a **sensory integration hub** and receives:

- Vagal input from the gut

- Signals about gastric distension

- Visceral sensory information

- Cardiovascular inputs

From the NTS, GLP-1–producing neurons project out onto the rest of the brain widely.

Where GLP-1 Receptors Are Located

Given that GLP-1 is made in the NTS, where does it have its effects in the brain? To examine this, we need to look for where GLP-1 receptors are found throughout the brain. High-density regions of these receptors include the hypothalamus (particularly the arcuate nucleus and paraventricular nucleus), the area postrema, the NTS itself, the ventral tegmental area, nucleus accumbens, and the amygdala.

This distribution is striking because it means GLP-1 signaling intersects with:

- Appetite regulation

- Reward circuitry

- Stress responses

- Autonomic tone (automatic processes to maintain the body's physiology)

- Nausea pathways

So GLP-1 receptors are not confined to "hunger centers". They are also embedded in motivational circuits, stress responses and the maintenance of normal physiology.

Projection Map in the Brain

Target	Function
Hypothalamic PVN & ARC	Integrates with leptin/insulin/melanocortin systems → appetite, energy expenditure
Amygdala & BNST	Anxiety, conditioned taste aversion, "sickness" behaviors
Ventral tegmental area & nucleus accumbens	Dampens dopaminergic reward from food/drugs
Dorsal motor nucleus of vagus	Parasympathetic output → slows gastric emptying, lowers HR/BP

What Central GLP-1 Does

As we just saw, GLP-1 receptors are not confined to the brain's homeostatic centers. They are found in regions that shape motivation and reward, including the ventral tegmental area and nucleus accumbens, components of the mesolimbic dopamine system. These circuits help determine not only whether we are hungry, but how compelling food feels. They assign salience and encode desire.

Experimental work in animals shows that activating GLP-1 receptors in these regions reduces the motivation to obtain highly palatable food. Conditioned responses weaken and the drive to pursue reward softens. In some models, GLP-1 signaling alters dopaminergic activity itself, not eliminating reward, but modulating its intensity.

In humans, neuroimaging studies suggest a similar pattern: GLP-1 receptor activation reduces anticipatory responses to food cues. The brain's reaction to the promise of food changes. Cravings shift even before the first bite. This is not simply delayed gastric emptying but altered valuation. GLP-1 in the brain recalibrates how much reward is assigned to intake, signaling fullness and impacting desire. Under physiologic conditions, this modulation is brief and contextual, tied to meals, to visceral input, and to transient states. Rising and falling, it refines appetite without erasing it.

Understanding this central circuitry is essential because when GLP-1 signaling becomes sustained rather than episodic, it is these motivational networks that are continuously engaged.

Homeostatic Hunger vs. Hedonic Motivation

Not all hunger is the same. We'll look at two types of hunger here. A third type, called Hidden Hunger, will be discussed in a later chapter.

Homeostatic hunger is the body's signal that energy is required. This hunger arises from metabolic need signaled by falling glucose, rising ghrelin (a hormone that stimulates appetite and hunger sensations), and depleted glycogen. It is regulated primarily in hypothalamic centers of the brain that monitor fuel status and maintain survival.

Hedonic motivation is the desire to eat in the presence of abundance. This hunger is not driven by deficit but by valuation, social/environmental cues, anticipation, and learned association. A person can be physiologically full and still feel compelled by dessert. These two systems overlap but are not identical.

Homeostatic hunger answers the question: *Do I need energy?* Hedonic motivation addresses: *How rewarding would this be?* And GLP-1 intersects with both.

In the hypothalamus, GLP-1 signaling influences energy balance and satiety, modulating homeostatic intake. In the ventral tegmental area and nucleus accumbens, GLP-1 receptor activation influences reward valuation, modulating hedonic drive. This dual placement doesn't merely close the metabolic ledger, it adjusts the perceived value of consumption.

Under physiologic conditions, this modulation is proportional and transient. After a meal, reward sensitivity to further eating diminishes and the system recalibrates. The desire to eat fades. As blood glucose starts to drop, appetite returns appropriately. That rhythm preserves flexibility.

When GLP-1 signaling becomes sustained rather than episodic, it is not only metabolic hunger that changes. When we speak of appetite suppression, we mean altered neural valuation, not just delayed gastric emptying. Feeding motivation shifts toward a lowered reward expectation. As you will see in the next section, long-acting GLP-1 receptor drugs cross the blood–brain barrier to varying degrees and have prolonged access to central GLP-1 receptors. To those who experience a lot of "food noise" (constant stimulation and thoughts of food), GLP-1 in the brain modulates how compelling food feels, and this, is the ultimate game changer.

Enter Pharmacologic Amplification

In the early 1990s, Dr. John Eng, a researcher at the VA Medical Center in the Bronx, NY, was studying the saliva of a lizard called the Gila monster

(*Heloderma suspectum*). Its venom caused enlargement in the pancreas of mice, and he wondered if it might influence insulin production. He isolated the peptide which was named exendin-4 and found that it bound to the GLP-1 receptor. Even more fortuitously, it resisted rapid degradation by DPP-4, which made it a possible drug target for diabetes. In 2005, exenatide, the synthetic version of exendin-4, was approved for glucose control in Type 2 Diabetes (DM2).

The science so far: GLP-1 enhances insulin secretion in a glucose-dependent manner, lowers after-meal glucose, and reduces A1C, a measure of average blood sugar levels over 2-3 months. Weight loss was observed, but secondarily. The focus at this point was blood sugar control.

Over time, newer molecules followed, modified to extend the half-life, and hence the duration of drug effects. These are not identical to your body's GLP-1 and were specifically engineered for persistence. Native GLP-1 lasts minutes while the synthetic products last days. Native GLP-1 is released in a pulsatile fashion; the drugs provide sustained receptor occupancy. This difference is not trivial as it changes the rhythm of signaling.

From Diabetes to Obesity

As mentioned above, the early trials focused on glycemic endpoints, followed by cardiovascular outcome trials. But soon, the weight-loss effect grew harder to ignore.

Higher doses were tested, pushing for greater weight loss effects. In 2021, semaglutide was approved for chronic weight management and the world of obesity medicine was inundated with questions and demand. Media coverage hyped it, celebrities sought access, clinics multiplied, and prescriptions surged. What began as a diabetes therapy was now a cultural phenomenon.

It seemed that science and technology had triumphed in the most dramatic and impactful way. With these new drugs, obesity would soon be a thing of the past and its associated diseases and health risks would decline significantly. Traditional and social media, influencers, and bio-hackers proclaimed that GLP-1 was a "natural hormone" made in the gut to help control weight and for many, the assumption that it was "made in our bodies" meant it was safe. But there are important differences between our body's GLP-1 system and pharmacological intervention.

Physiologic vs. Pharmacologic Doses

When weight loss effects were noted with diabetic doses of GLP-1 drugs, the natural question was: what if we raised the dose? Bear in mind that diabetic doses are already above what your physiology is designed to handle (i.e., supraphysiologic). Here's a look at your native GLP-1 levels vs. various drug levels:

Item	Typical steady-state blood level	Fold vs physiologic peak (10 pmol/L)	Fold vs physiologic fasting (2 pmol/L)
Physiologic intact GLP-1 (fasting)	<2 pmol/L	—	—
Physiologic intact GLP-1 (post-meal peak)	5–10 pmol/L	—	—
Oral semaglutide (Wegovy tablets 25 mg daily)	~77 nmol/L	~7,700×	~38,500×
Tirzepatide 5 mg weekly (calc.)	~110 nmol/L	~11,041×	~55,205×
Tirzepatide 10 mg weekly (calc.)	~221 nmol/L	~22,082×	~110,410×
Tirzepatide 15 mg weekly (calc.)	~331 nmol/L	~33,123×	~165,615×

Let's walk though it together to understand the implications of these dosing levels.

When you first look at these numbers, the difference appears almost implausible. Physiologic intact GLP-1 peaks at roughly 5–10 pmol/L after a meal and falls back toward baseline within minutes. The pharmacologic agents circulate in the range of tens to hundreds of nanomoles per liter. A nanomole is 1,000 picomoles, so 77 nmol/L is 77,000 pmol/L, and 110 nmol/L is 110,000 pmol/L. At face value, this appears to represent thousands to tens of thousands of times higher circulating concentrations than endogenous GLP-1.

However, those values represent total drug in plasma, and the receptor does not see total drug. It sees free drug, or **unbound** drug levels.

Bound vs. Unbound

Long-acting GLP-1 receptor drugs were deliberately engineered to bind to a ubiquitous plasma protein called albumin. That is how their half-life is extended from minutes to days. For semaglutide and tirzepatide (a combination GLP-1 + GIP drug), more than 99% of the circulating drug is albumin-bound at steady state. The unbound fraction is typically on the order of **0.1–0.3%**.

Only the unbound fraction can freely diffuse to receptors, making it biologically active. So the conceptual correction is simple: Free concentration ≈ Total concentration × Unbound fraction. If we take oral semaglutide at ~77 nmol/L total, that equals 77–230 pmol/L free drug (0.1-0,3%)

Now compare that to physiologic intact GLP-1 where peak active GLP-1 ≈ 5–10 pmol/L. Even after correcting for albumin binding, free semaglutide drug levels are still plausibly **7–40× higher than physiologic peaks**, and dramatically higher than fasting baseline.

For tirzepatide at 110–331 nmol/L total, even applying the same 0.1–0.3% free fraction yields free concentrations in the 100–1,000+ pmol/L range, which would represent **an order of magnitude or more above physiologic peak levels.** So while the "thousands-fold" numbers shrink once binding is accounted for, it remains meaningfully **supraphysiologic**. Most importantly we are talking about continuous elevation of the hormone.

Continuous Receptor Occupancy

Under physiologic conditions, GLP-1 receptor activation is intermittent. Under pharmacologic dosing, receptors are occupied continuously.

This has several consequences:

- Appetite suppression becomes sustained
- Gastric emptying remains slowed
- Glucagon tone is chronically modulated
- Energy intake decreases persistently

The body is no longer responding to a meal. It is responding to a **constant signal**.

Biological systems rely on fluctuation. Insulin rises and falls; cortisol rises and falls. Sympathetic tone, native GLP-1, leptin and ghrelin all oscillate and cycle through the day. This rhythmic rise and ebb permits sensitivity, allowing receptors to downregulate, and feedback loops to recalibrate and compensate.

Receptor Occupancy — Why It's Hard to Calculate

Concentration alone does not equal receptor activation. To estimate receptor occupancy, we need:

- Free drug concentration
- The drug's binding affinity (Kd) for the GLP-1 receptor
- Tissue distribution
- Receptor density
- On/off kinetics

While we can approximate that pharmacologic dosing produces substantially higher and more sustained receptor engagement than physiologic pulses, precise occupancy in human tissues is not directly measurable.

The Deeper Difference: Pulse vs Plateau

Physiologic ('natural') GLP-1 occurs in brief spikes with rapid degradation, intermittent receptor activation, and a clear on–off rhythm. In contrast, pharmacologic GLP-1 RAs (drugs) provide sustained steady-state plasma levels, continuous receptor engagement, and minimal return to baseline between meals.

Even if free concentrations were only modestly higher than peak physiologic levels, the area under the curve over 24 hours measuring the body's total exposure to the drug over time, is dramatically greater. This is not merely about amplitude but also duration. Biologic systems evolved under oscillation. Sustained signaling alters adaptation.

So What Are We Modifying?

When we compare physiologic and pharmacologic exposure, we are not simply increasing a hormone that was deficient. We are:

- Elevating baseline GLP-1 receptor tone
- Extending its duration from minutes to days
- Increasing receptor occupancy above meal-triggered peaks
- Removing the natural troughs that restore sensitivity

The table reminds us that synthetic GLP-1 receptor agonists are not replacements for a missing pulse but act as sustained amplifiers of a signal that was designed to be transient.

Shifts in Allocation

GLP-1 receptor agonists reduce energy intake, creating a negative energy balance. Weight and fat mass decline, as does lean mass (up to 30-40% of the weight lost with GLP-1 drugs is from lean mass loss). Due to appetite suppression, food–and, therefore, nutrient–intake may decrease. The inhibition of glucagon by GLP-1 may alter the liver-alpha cell axis and amino acid flux may shift.

These are not neutral changes and affect more than just body weight. Synthetic does not mean "identical"; the drugs are not merely replacing a missing hormone but are amplifying one branch of a coordinated network. And when we alter synchrony, duration, and rhythm, we alter architecture.

Side Effects as Signals

Reports in the media have familiarized us with the common adverse effects of GLP-1 drugs: nausea, vomiting, diarrhea, and early satiety. These are understandable extensions of slowed gastric emptying and central appetite signaling. But other questions remain open:

- With GLP-1 inhibiting glucagon secretion, how does chronic suppression of glucagon affect amino acid economy?

- What happens to alpha-cell signaling over years?

- How does sustained central GLP-1 tone alter neural circuits?

- How does immune signaling adapt?

- What happens when the drug is withdrawn?

Now that these drugs have entered mainstream medicine, these are naturally the next layer of inquiry we should subject them to.

Domain	Endogenous GLP-1 (Axis)	GLP-1 Receptor Agonists (Drugs)
Primary Source	Intestinal L-cells (ileum > colon); NTS / brainstem neurons	Synthetic peptides or analogues injected or oral; delivered systemically
Pattern of Exposure	Short-lived, pulsatile release tied to meals, microbiota signals, IL-6, and circadian rhythm	Sustained, supraphysiologic receptor stimulation, often weeks-long
Main Physiologic Actions	Fine-tuned: glucose-dependent insulin secretion; transient glucagon suppression; slowed gastric emptying; satiety; local immune modulation	Potent: large, durable appetite suppression; strong glucagon suppression; marked delays in gastric emptying; weight loss; off-target immune and neuroendocrine effects
Integration with Other Proglucagon Products	Secreted alongside oxyntomodulin, glicentin, GLP-2; acts in concert with glucagon and GIP	Pharmacologic signal often decoupled from normal proglucagon constellation and from physiologic glucagon rhythms
Role in Metabolic Balance	Coordinates nutrient inflow with insulin, liver metabolism, gut integrity, and immune status; responds to acute stress/infection	Drives weight loss and glycemic control by overriding appetite and glucagon physiology; may destabilize protein economy and immune balance in some contexts
Temporal Logic	Designed for short-term, reversible responses (meals, acute illness, transient inflammation)	Used for chronic, often open-ended therapy in heterogeneous immune/metabolic states
Context Sensitivity	Highly sensitive to microbiota, IL 6, circadian timing, sex, age, and tissue state	Same dose in very different biological contexts; trials rarely stratify by immune state, microbiota, or lean-mass risk
Clinical	Subtle: postprandial glucose	Visible: dramatic weight loss, GI

Phenotype	control, modest satiety, gut repair; largely invisible unless failing	symptoms, sometimes nausea, fatigue, body-composition shifts, and immune-mediated events

Comparison Table Between Physiologic and Pharmacologic GLP-1

Bottom Line

The proglucagon system is a coordinated metabolic governance network.

GLP-1 drugs:

- Increase signal amplitude
- Extend signal duration
- Elevate baseline receptor tone
- Reduce physiologic oscillation

The question is not whether they work but rather how sustained modification of a pulsatile system reshapes the architecture over time.

****

Chapter 3

It started with furniture. When I was in residency training, my then-husband, M, was still in engineering school. We were both first-generation immigrants trying to establish a life in the US.

Boston is not only defined by the seasons but also its universities and colleges. Life in the city is held hostage on two dreaded days: Move-in Day and its equally migrainous counterpart, Move-out Day. Streets are blocked off by moving trucks driven by hungover students, and parking, already a scarcity, becomes non-existent. Bostonians' experiences of these days range from bewilderment and frustration to knowing smiles and resigned forbearance, depending on how long one has lived in the city. The only festivity to come out of this mess is a phenomenon known as Storrowing, when a moving truck gets stuck as it tries to go under low-clearance bridges along Storrow Drive. Most sightings occur at the Old CSX Rail Bridge near the BU Bridge and the Harvard Street Bridge. Seasoned Bostonians, wise enough not to drive on such a day, watch as they stroll along the Charles River, or on their TV screens. It's a sight guaranteed to cheer even the most winter-grinched hearts.

The scourge of Move-out Day is mitigated by one other thing–free stuff. That it is mostly beer-stained, funky-smelling free stuff does not thwart the enthusiasm of dumpster divers and bargain hunters (what could be a better bargain than free?). My ex ditched the Salvation Army after his first Move-out forage. We eventually filled our home with a slipcovered sagging couch (the sides were still quite firm), a picnic table (real wood) in the kitchen, an armchair and side tables, and an old stationary bike that was my cardio workhorse throughout residency.

But then our space started filling up with stuff we had no need for. An old, non-functioning wood-stove, a battered golf bag with two golf clubs (neither of us played), a toy kitchen set. Because we lived in one half of an old townhouse (rent reduced because I painted all of its interior and we were okay with extra-extra-shabby-bordering-on-dingy chic), he had half a basement to store his finds. Within weeks, it was unnavigable. At the time I was unaware of hoarding behavior, and it became an exhausting pattern of cleaning out and organizing, only to have the space fill up again with more stuff, followed by yet more decluttering. Purge, binge, purge, binge. It's no coincidence that food binges involve stuffing, and stuff purges end in dumps.

Strongest predictors of hoarding tendencies seem to be childhood scarcity and trauma. My fellow medical residents from the former Soviet Union were overwhelmed by supermarkets. Sixteen types of honey, eighteen brands of toilet paper, fresh meat, canned meat, frozen, dried, and even freeze-dried varieties. Picking out a carton of milk turned out to be almost equivalent in complexity to Soviet bureaucracy. And it wasn't just food. It was clothing and cars, bedsheets, doormats, pens, printers, and postage stamps (the *Red Sox Nation* series or *Dog Breeds of the World*?).

M could not walk away from anything put out on the sidewalk. Even if it was broken he was handy enough to resuscitate it, and if he wasn't, he liked to think that in the future, he would find a way to repair it. While I didn't do much scavenging, once an object was brought into the house, I had a hard time 'turning it out.' It felt like an act of abandonment. So while it started as a creative way to live frugally, it became emblematic of a way of relating to the world we were thrust in. We were both from middle-class families, so scarcity was not a fundamental issue here.

But we were unprepared for an America that was at once the ambered land of Plenty and vast inner plains fruited with Empty.

It is tempting to describe these medications as if they simply correct a missing signal or replace a hormone the body lacks. But obesity is not a straightforward hormone deficiency, and GLP-1 drugs are not simple replacement therapy. They act on appetite, glucose regulation, gut signaling, reward, inflammation, energy balance, and weight regulation within a dynamic system that is already adapting, defending, and responding.

This chapter examines what happens when we move beyond GLP-1 alone and begin combining hormonal signals from the same biological family. Dual and triple agonists may produce greater weight loss, but they also raise deeper questions: which pathways are being amplified, which family dynamics are being altered, and what kind of weight is actually being lost?

GLP-1 Resistance in Type 2 Diabetes

In healthy physiology, the incretin system is anticipatory. When nutrients enter the gut, intestinal L-cells release GLP-1. The level rises quickly, peaks modestly, and falls within minutes. It enhances glucose-stimulated insulin secretion, tempers glucagon release, slows gastric emptying, and communicates satiety to the brain. We've already seen that it is not a dominant hormone but a contextual one.

In DM2 (type 2 diabetes), the incretin effect is impaired. Normally, insulin secretion that follows eating sugar is amplified by incretins such as GLP-1, but with diabetes this is reduced. β-cells respond less robustly and glucagon suppression becomes erratic. The system is distorted, with altered central satiety signaling. This distortion has been described as "GLP-1 deficiency," a poor word choice as what is happening isn't deficiency of the hormone in the true sense. Anyone using GLP-1 deficiency to explain it is misunderstanding the mechanism at work.

In many individuals with obesity and Type 2 diabetes, GLP-1 is still produced. It may even rise after meals. **What changes is the responsiveness of the system**. The β-cell becomes less sensitive. The α-cell becomes less appropriately restrained. The brain's appetite circuitry may not interpret the signal with the same fidelity. This decrease in responsiveness is called resistance.

Pharmacologic GLP-1 receptor agonists enter this landscape at concentrations far beyond physiologic pulses. They do not restore the subtle, meal-linked rise-and-fall of endogenous GLP-1. Instead they impose a sustained receptor signal resulting in improvement of blood sugar levels, lowering of glucagon levels and a decline in appetite. This is done not by restoring the system but **through an override of a partially resistant system**.

Understanding that distinction is essential if we are to evaluate both the benefits and the boundaries of long-term pharmacologic incretin signaling.

Are GLP-1 Levels Lower in Obesity?

Several studies have examined whether individuals with obesity produce less GLP-1 after meals. A 2019 study (doi: 10.3889/oamjms.2019.030) compared GLP-1 responses in individuals with obesity and those without.

The findings were not dramatic. GLP-1 was present in both groups and differences, where observed, were modest. In some analyses, statistical significance was limited. The data did not demonstrate absence of GLP-1 secretion, suggesting variability instead.

Obesity is often described in public discourse as a "GLP-1 deficiency." But deficiency implies something specific: a consistent, reproducible hormonal absence that explains disease. The evidence does not show that. Even when post-meal GLP-1 responses are somewhat lower in obesity, several questions remain unresolved:

- Does lower GLP-1 precede weight gain, or follow it?
- Is production reduced, or is the breakdown process altered?
- Does receptor responsiveness change?
- Does weight loss restore GLP-1 dynamics?

In many individuals, weight loss, particularly after bariatric surgery, enhances postprandial GLP-1 responses substantially. Caloric restriction alone can modify incretin signaling. That plasticity argues against a fixed primary deficiency state.

GLP-1 tone doesn't disappear but shifts with metabolic context. Calling obesity a "GLP-1 deficiency" therefore oversimplifies a far more dynamic system.

What Counts as a Hormone Deficiency?

In endocrinology, the term *deficiency* carries specific meaning. It generally requires:

- Consistently reduced hormone levels below established physiologic range
- Reproducibility across large cohorts
- A clinical phenotype directly attributable to low levels
- Restoration of physiology with physiologic replacement dosing
- Intact receptor responsiveness

Classic examples include insulin deficiency in Type 1 diabetes or cortisol deficiency in Addison's disease.

To label obesity a state of GLP-1 deficiency, we would need to demonstrate sustained, reproducible absence of GLP-1 signaling that precedes weight gain and normalizes with physiologic (not supraphysiologic) replacement. Current evidence does not meet that threshold.

A Broken Receptor ≠ Missing Hormone

The idea of "GLP-1 deficiency" has gained traction in part because of how a genetic study led by Michael Lutter has been discussed publicly. The study itself did not show that common obesity is caused by a lack of GLP-1. Rather, it identified rare variants affecting neuropeptide signaling, including variants that may impair GLP-1 receptor signaling. That distinction is crucial as a receptor signaling defect is not the same thing as hormone deficiency.

The study is valuable in that it confirms that intact GLP-1 receptor signaling contributes to metabolic regulation. However, it does not demonstrate that common obesity is caused by GLP-1 deficiency. A hormone is part of a signaling pathway: secretion from one tissue, circulation through blood, binding to a receptor, intracellular cascades, gene transcription, feedback loops. When any part of that pathway becomes less responsive, we call it a signaling defect or resistance. In that case, the problem is not the absence of the signal but defective transmission. A rare receptor mutation is categorically different from a population-level hormonal deficit, and the rarity of these variants highlights how uncommon true receptor-level disruption is.

Imagine a light switch connected to a lamp. If the wiring in the wall is damaged, pressing the switch harder will not fix the problem. The issue is not insufficient pressure on the switch; the problem is faulty circuitry. You can flip the switch repeatedly, even apply greater force, but if the electrical pathway is compromised, the bulb will not light up.

The rare GLP-1 receptor variants described in the Lutter study are examples of signaling defects. The receptor itself does not transmit the message efficiently. In that situation, the problem is not that too little GLP-1 is present. The problem lies in the receptor's ability to respond. Increasing the amount of hormone does not repair a defective receptor. At most, higher concentrations may partially force residual signaling through whatever function remains. That is amplification, not correction.

Genetic signaling defects should not be invoked as proof of hormone deficiency. A rare GLP-1 receptor variant is like faulty wiring. It tells us the circuit matters but does not prove the room is dark because there is no electricity. A broken receptor is not the same as a missing hormone, and more hormone is not the same as fixing the circuitry.

Pharmacologic Override

If obesity is not a simple state of GLP-1 deficiency, and rare receptor defects are not corrected by more GLP-1, then what exactly are GLP-1 receptor agonists doing? They are not "replacing a missing hormone". Instead **they impose a sustained receptor signal**.

We've already seen that endogenous GLP-1 is released in brief pulses after meals. It rises modestly and is rapidly degraded. The signal is contextual and transient. GLP-1 drugs circulate continuously, their concentrations exceeding physiologic peaks by orders of magnitude. Receptor occupancy is sustained rather than meal-linked.

In DM2, glycemic control improves as appetite declines and glucagon secretion falls. These effects are clinically meaningful. For many patients, they are transformative. But the mechanism is not restoration of a lost physiologic rhythm. **It is an override of a partially resistant network.** Essentially, we're turning up the volume in a sound system because the speakers are damaged.

Override can be therapeutic in that it can compensate for defective signaling and restore functional outputs, leading to lower glucose, reduced energy intake, and weight loss. Yet override also changes the character of the system. A signal that was once pulsatile becomes continuous. A feedback loop that once oscillated around meals now experiences persistent receptor engagement. The question is not whether this works in the short term but what sustained override does to the larger endocrine architecture.

We will return later to this issue in a later chapter when we discuss metabolic adaptation and rebound physiology. For now, it is enough to recognize that pharmacologic incretin therapy amplifies signaling far beyond physiologic replacement. That distinction becomes even more important when combination therapies enter the picture.

Combination Agonists: Recomposing Endocrine Axes

The next generation of therapies not only amplifies GLP-1, it also recruits other hormones.

Dual and triple agonists pair GLP-1 with other peptides such as glucagon (same biological family) or GIP (in-laws). These hormones evolved to counterbalance one another across feeding and fasting states. They pulse, rise, and fall within tightly regulated contexts. Combination drugs alter that choreography.

GLP-1 suppresses glucagon in many settings. Yet some dual agonists include glucagon receptor activity with GLP-1 action. GIP has distinct effects on metabolism and fat. When these pathways are stimulated simultaneously and continuously, the endocrine system no longer oscillates in its usual pattern. Though not inherently harmful as far as we know, we should note that it alters physiology.

The body regulates energy through **counter-regulation** — insulin and glucagon, feeding and fasting, storage and mobilization. Combination agonists compress those distinctions into a single, sustained pharmacologic signal. In doing so, they may produce greater weight loss and improved glycemia. They may also reshape nutrient handling in the liver, amino-acid flux, and pancreatic feedback loops in ways that have not yet been fully characterized.

To understand those downstream consequences, we must examine one of the key regulatory circuits affected by glucagon signaling: the liver–α-cell axis. That axis is where sustained suppression — or recombination — of glucagon signaling impacts physiology.

Re-enter The Liver–α-Cell Axis

Glucagon is often described simply as insulin's counter-hormone, a fasting signal that raises blood glucose. But as we've seen, its role is broader than glucose alone as it also regulates amino-acid metabolism.

To review: When amino acids rise after a protein-containing meal, they stimulate pancreatic α-cells to release glucagon. Glucagon then acts on the liver to promote amino-acid disposal, ureagenesis, and gluconeogenesis. As hepatic processing proceeds, circulating amino-acid levels fall, reducing α-cell stimulation. This feedback loop with amino acids stimulating glucagon, glucagon promoting hepatic amino-acid clearance, forms what is now recognized as the liver–α-cell axis.

When glucagon signaling is impaired at the receptor level, experimental models show a predictable pattern: circulating amino acids rise. Persistently elevated amino acids stimulate α-cells. Over time, α-cell mass can expand — a phenomenon termed α-cell hyperplasia (ACH). In some animal models involving profound and sustained glucagon receptor blockade, reactive α-cell hyperplasia has progressed further, occasionally toward pancreatic neuroendocrine changes. These findings have shaped our understanding of glucagon's roles in growth and metabolic regulation.

Importantly, GLP-1 receptor agonists do not eliminate glucagon signaling. They suppress glucagon secretion, particularly in hyperglycemic states (and in some studies, with normoglycemia). This suppression is sustained relative to normal physiologic oscillation and it raises a question.

If chronic glucagon receptor blockade can alter the liver–α-cell feedback loop, what are the long-term implications of sustained glucagon suppression? Does the axis remain stable? Does hepatic amino-acid handling adapt? Are there contexts in which feedback becomes exaggerated? At present, we do not have definitive answers.

Large clinical trials have not demonstrated clear, consistent increases in pancreatic cancer attributed to GLP-1 drugs, and regulatory reviews over the past decade have not established causation. Yet emerging signals, including recent regulatory cautions regarding possible fatal pancreatic inflammation, remind us that endocrine systems are interconnected. When we modulate incretin tone chronically, we are not only influencing appetite and glycemia. We are also altering glucagon dynamics, hepatic nutrient handling, and pancreatic feedback circuits.

Whether these alterations remain fully adaptive over years of sustained drug exposure is a scientific question that warrants careful study.

Emerging Signals and the Question of α-Cell Hyperplasia

In February 2026, a News Explainer in Nature summarized recent regulatory communications from the United Kingdom and Brazil regarding a possible association between GLP-1 receptor agonists and pancreatic inflammation. The article emphasized that causality has not been established. Large randomized trials have not demonstrated a clear, reproducible increase in pancreatitis or pancreatic cancer attributed to these agents. Nevertheless, regulators acknowledged that signals in drug vigilance data warrant continued monitoring. Such signals do not prove harm but they do invite mechanistic scrutiny. To understand why, we return to the liver–α-cell axis.

In animal models in which glucagon receptor signaling is profoundly reduced (either through genetic knockout or sustained pharmacologic blockade) a predictable sequence has been observed. Circulating amino acids rise and α-cells experience persistent growth stimulation. Over time, α-cell hyperplasia (increase in the number of α-cells) develops. In some long-duration models of near-complete glucagon receptor blockade, proliferative changes have extended further, occasionally toward pancreatic neuroendocrine tumor formation.

These findings do not demonstrate that GLP-1 receptor agonists cause α-cell hyperplasia in humans. GLP-1 therapies suppress glucagon; they do not abolish receptor signaling. But the animal data clarify a principle: the pancreas responds to sustained alterations in glucagon signaling.

α-cells are not static. They adapt to nutrient flux and receptor tone. When amino-acid disposal through the liver is impaired, feedback drives expansion. When signaling balance is restored, the axis recalibrates. GLP-1 receptor agonists do not replicate glucagon receptor knockout. The question is whether sustained pharmacologic incretin tone, particularly when combined with other agonists as in the combo drugs, shifts the liver–α-cell feedback program in subtle ways over years of exposure.

If α-cell hyperplasia were to occur in a clinical setting, potential risks would include:

- Altered glucagon dynamics
- Disrupted amino-acid handling
- Increased endocrine cell mass with theoretical cancer growth risk
- Paracrine effects within the pancreas affecting exocrine tissue

These are hypotheses grounded in experimental biology, not yet established or disproved in clinical outcomes.

At present, human data remain reassuring overall though long-term endocrine remodeling is difficult to detect early. Pancreatic imaging lacks the resolution to identify modest α-cell expansion and subtle changes in amino-acid economy may go unmeasured in routine care. Do chronic incretin therapies alter hepatic amino-acid flux? Do glucagon dynamics shift over time? Are there subgroups — such as individuals with chronic kidney disease, altered protein metabolism, or pre-existing glucagon dysregulation — in whom the axis behaves differently?

The liver–α-cell axis reminds us that endocrine systems are reciprocal. When we modulate one node chronically, feedback circuits adapt. Whether those adaptations remain fully benign over decades of therapy is a matter for careful longitudinal study.

Combination Agonists: Promise and Compression of Physiology

Dual and triple agonists such as GLP-1/GIP agents and GLP-1/GIP/glucagon combinations are designed to produce greater weight loss and metabolic improvement than GLP-1 alone. The strategy was not merely to increase signal amplitude, but to reshape signal geometry. By activating multiple receptors simultaneously, combination therapies may overcome partial resistance within any single pathway. They may also more closely mimic the complex hormonal milieu seen after bariatric surgery, where GLP-1, GIP, PYY, and other peptides rise together.

The potential advantages include greater weight loss, improved blood sugar control, enhanced insulin sensitivity, with possible improvements in lipid profiles. From a clinical standpoint, this can translate into dramatic reductions in weight and HbA1c.

Dual Agonists: GLP-1/GIP

In normal physiology, GIP and GLP-1 are temporally staggered signals. GIP is released early from K-cells in the duodenum and proximal jejunum as nutrients first enter the small intestine. It promotes insulin secretion and facilitates nutrient storage, particularly in fat tissue. Historically, GIP was considered "ineffective" in DM2 due to resistance. The dual-agonist strategy is likely based on high-potency GIPR (GIP Receptor) stimulation to overcome resistance, similar to GLP-1R override. Simultaneous GLP-1R activation may also restore β-cell responsiveness to GIP.

GIP receptor agonism may improve insulin sensitivity due to increased glucose uptake into fat tissue for storage in the form of triacyl-glycerols or triglycerides and prevents the spillage of toxic free fatty acids into the blood. This helps reduce visceral, hepatic, and other ectopic lipid deposition. GIP may also enhance glucagon secretion when blood glucose is low or normal. This may counter the inhibitory effect of GLP-1 on glucagon secretion. In the central nervous system, GIP hypothalamic signaling may reduce food intake, enhancing GLP-1's anorectic effect. More significantly, it may reduce GLP-1-associated nausea, improving tolerability and adherence.

The important caveat to this is that physiologically, unhealthy diet-driven GIP production leads to fat storage and, when hypersecreted, possibly visceral and hepatic lipid accumulation. Thus, GIP is metabolically double-edged: protective when adipose tissue is acting as a competent buffer, but potentially contributing when nutrient excess, adipose dysfunction, and chronic hyperglycemia distort that buffering role.

Early (GIP) signal→ "prepare to store"

Later (GLP-1) signal→ "slow intake and regulate output"

This staggered choreography allows coordinated energy handling across the length of the gut. In dual GLP-1/GIP agonist therapy, that temporal sequencing is removed. Both receptors are stimulated continuously and simultaneously, independent of nutrient progression. The physiologic "early-then-late" rhythm becomes a sustained composite signal.

There are also current studies for the development of combination agents with GLP-1 agonist and GIP antagonist. Physiologically GIP antagonism blocks the fat-storing properties of GIP, thereby augmenting the GLP-1 agonist effect. Both GIP agonism and antagonism with GLP-1 agents provide greater weight loss effects through different pathways and mechanisms.

Trade-offs and Open Questions

With dual agonist drugs such as tirzepatide, sustained dual incretin stimulation further compresses physiologic oscillation. Chronic GIPR activation in adipose tissue raises questions about long-term adipocyte biology while glucagon dynamics may differ relative to GLP-1 monotherapy. In short, the therapeutic gain is potency while the biologic cost is deeper network modification.

Triple Agonists: GLP-1/GIP/Glucagon

These agents attempt to integrate appetite suppression (GLP-1), insulinotropic enhancement and nausea abatement (GIP), and energy expenditure increase (glucagon). The design logic is tolerance and efficiency, addressing intake, expenditure and insulin resistance simultaneously. The trial results show dramatic weight reduction and glycemic control.

Mechanistic Considerations

Triple agonism represents maximal endocrine compression:

- Simultaneous sustained activation of three receptors
- Continuous signaling across feeding and fasting axes
- Deep engagement of hepatic, pancreatic, adipose, and central circuits

The potential advantages are substantial metabolic efficacy but they amplify both opportunity and uncertainty, leading to the following biologic questions:

- How does chronic GCGR activation intersect with LACA (Liver-Alpha-Cell-Axis) over years?
- Does triple receptor occupancy alter tissue-specific desensitization patterns?
- What is the long-term lean mass trajectory under simultaneous anorectic and catabolic drive?

Physiologic Considerations

In normal metabolic cycles the different gut hormones counterbalance each other across time. Combination drugs compress these oscillations into sustained, overlapping stimulation.

When GLP-1 tends towards suppression of glucagon while a co-agonist stimulates the glucagon receptor, the system is no longer cycling through fasting–feeding counter-regulation. It is receiving a composite signal that does not fully exist in nature. Adding just GLP-1 alone is like adding 3 tubas to the usual 1 in an orchestra and drowning out the other sections. With combination therapy, we are adding 3 tubas, 6 trumpets *and* 5 trombones to the orchestra. This changes feedback and physiologic settings in our body and distorts its inherent music.

Questions Raised by Combination Therapy

- Does sustained multi-receptor activation alter long-term endocrine adaptation?

- How does chronic glucagon receptor engagement interact with hepatic amino-acid handling?

- Does combining anorectic and catabolic signals shift muscle mass preservation?

- Are feedback circuits given time to recalibrate, or are they held in continuous drive?

Combination therapy may represent a development in potency. It may also represent increasing endocrine compression with fewer rhythmic pulses and more constancy, like a doorbell that keeps ringing and never stops. Whether that constancy remains benign over decades is not yet known.

Oral Semaglutide: Expanding Access, Altering Exposure

Injectable GLP-1 receptor agonists create relatively stable systemic exposure over days to weeks. Some people have avoided the GLP-1 drugs because they cannot tolerate injections. The oral formulation of semaglutide represents a different kind of innovation by changing the mode of delivery. Oral semaglutide, formulated with an absorption enhancer, allows peptide delivery through a pill.

Potential Advantages

- Improved patient acceptance
- Elimination of injections
- Earlier treatment adoption
- Expanded global access

For many patients, the psychological barrier of injection is overcome but oral delivery introduces different pharmacokinetic characteristics.

Physiologic Considerations

Oral semaglutide requires:

- Strict fasting conditions
- Limited water intake
- Delayed food consumption after dosing

Absorption can be variable. Blood levels may fluctuate depending on how closely you follow dosing instructions. Unlike your native GLP-1 which rises in response to meals, oral semaglutide produces receptor engagement independent of nutrient context. The signal precedes food intake and persists beyond meal-related physiology. In that sense, oral therapy does not restore natural incretin timing and maintains the pharmacologic override model. At the highest dose, oral semaglutide can potentially produce weight loss results equivalent to the injectable drugs (mean loss of 33 lbs–37.4 lbs over 1 ¼ years.)

Questions Raised by Oral Delivery

- Does variable absorption produce fluctuating receptor occupancy?

- Does the stomach lining alter local signaling of the drug?

- How does chronic gastric absorption compare with subcutaneous systemic delivery in long-term tissue distribution?

Physiology vs. Control Theory: The Danger of a Fixed Output

Physiology is not merely a collection of pathways but a living system of feedback.

In the body, signals are rarely meant to stay loud forever. They rise and fall, amplify, quiet, and shift according to context. Insulin rises after a meal and falls when fasting. Inflammation activates in response to threat or injury, then ideally resolves. Appetite signals change with nutrient availability, gut distension, sleep, stress, illness, and energy need.

This is the body's intelligence. It adjusts inputs because conditions change. A signal that is useful in one context may become harmful in another if it is sustained too long, amplified too strongly, or uncoupled from feedback loops that regulate it. Physiology depends on timing, amplitude, location, sensitivity, and restraint.

Control theory offers a different system whereby the central concern is an output. A thermostat, for example, is designed to keep a room at a particular temperature. When the temperature falls below the set point, heat turns on. When the target is reached, heat turns off. The system compares the current state to the desired output and adjusts inputs to drive the output toward the target.

That logic is powerful but dangerous when applied too simplistically to biology. In medicine, we often become fixated on a desired output: lower glucose, lower blood pressure, lower LDL cholesterol, lower body weight. Once the output becomes the central goal, the temptation is to hard-lock the input that moves it. If one signal lowers the number, we sustain the signal. If more signal lowers the number further, we intensify it. If the output improves, we may assume the system has improved, but that is not how physiology works.

The body's own signaling systems are not usually loud, fixed, and continuous. They are dynamic and contextual, embedded in counter-signals, nutrient states, tissue needs, circadian timing, immune tone, stress responses, and repair demands. To take one signal and force it into a perpetual 'on' state because it produces the output we want is not the same thing as restoring physiology.

GLP-1 medications extend and amplify GLP-1 receptor signaling far beyond the body's normal temporal pattern which is precisely why they work. An 'always-on' GLP-1 signal can reduce appetite, alter food reward, slow gastric emptying, improve glycemia, and drive substantial weight loss. But the clinical question cannot stop at whether the output moved. The deeper question is: what happens when we hard-lock a signal for the sake of that output?

If the desired output is weight loss, we may become willing to keep appetite suppression loud and continuous. Yet appetite is not merely an inconvenience as it is connected to nutrient sufficiency, protein intake, muscle maintenance, immune function, bone health, mood, social eating, recovery, and long-term resilience. A medication that produces weight loss by suppressing intake may also reduce the signals that would normally protect against under-eating, under-protein intake, or loss of lean mass.

This is where physiology and control logic diverge. Physiology asks what the body needs now, and how signals should adjust. A fixed-output model asks what input keeps driving the number in a certain direction. Where physiology is responsive and adaptive, a hard-locked intervention can become rigid. The more forcefully we can move an output, the more carefully we have to ask what else is being moved, silenced, or reorganized along the way.

The danger in modern medicine is not that we use pharmacology. It is that we mistake pharmacologic control for physiologic restoration. A drug can help create the conditions for change. It can quiet food noise, reduce compulsive intake, improve glucose dynamics, and give a person enough space to rebuild patterns that were previously inaccessible. But if the only goal is to keep the weight-loss signal loud, then treatment becomes a kind of biological tunnel vision. We get the output we asked for, but not necessarily the health we intended.

Physiology vs. Control Theory

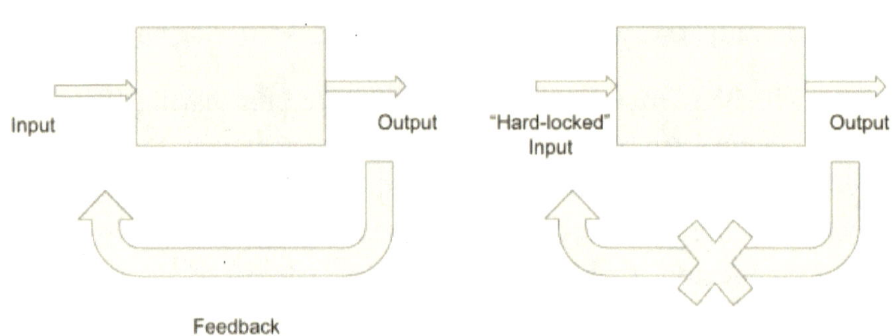

The central point of this section is not that combination drugs or oral semaglutide are dangerous. It is that as we increase potency and accessibility, we move further from physiologic rhythm and deeper into sustained, continuous receptor modulation.

In acute disease, override can be lifesaving and in chronic metabolic disease, override may even be transformative. But sustained multi-axis modulation invites long-term study. The more powerful the signal, the more carefully we must observe the system. Doorbells are useful and help us monitor when we have visitors. But when they ring incessantly, the sound begins to reshape our sleep, our mood, the home environment, and the way we live inside it.

Bottom Line

Common obesity is not a GLP-1 deficiency state. Evidence shows variability and context-dependence, not absence.

GLP-1 receptor agonists do not replace a missing hormone — they **override partially resistant signaling networks.**

Sustained pharmacologic receptor activation is different from physiologic pulsatility.

Combination drugs further compress, amplify and recombine endocrine axes that normally fluctuate in time in a balanced system.

Glucagon is part of a broader liver–α-cell feedback system regulating amino-acid metabolism, not just glucose. Profound disruption of this axis in animal models can lead to adaptive α-cell expansion (ACH), a reminder that endocrine systems remodel under chronic input.

Current human data are largely reassuring, but long-term, multi-axis modulation deserves structured surveillance, not assumption.

The central question: **What does sustained hormonal override do to metabolic governance over time?** (or what happens to you after living 8-10 years with a constantly ringing doorbell?)

****

Chapter 4

N's mother is from the Philippines and she is a hoarder. J's mother is from Haiti and she is a hoarder. E's father is from China and he is a hoarder. B's father has schizophrenia and is a hoarder.

It turns out that while hoarding occurs in 2-6% of the population, up to 20% of people exhibit sub-clinical hoarding behaviors, with immigrant and refugee populations showing more susceptibility to them. Scarcity and trauma leave scars. Migration amplifies this effect through economic insecurity, loss of cultural anchors, and hyper-frugality practices. People with hoarding disorder show difficulty deciding whether to discard items. Objects feel emotionally charged and discarding possessions actually activates distress signals in their brains.

I left home at 17, first for boarding school in England, and then for college in America. My friend, Monica, who had left for boarding school before me shared her best advice–*read everything and keep your ears open and you'll be okay*. So I read every sign, every article, every page, and listened to lectures, recordings, interviews of whatever it was I needed to learn. That was my main survival tool, not only for school, but all aspects of life. It never occurred to me to ask for help and the opposite happened instead.

I found myself unable to say no to anyone who needed my help. A friend couldn't make a car payment? I helped her out. M needed tuition for engineering school? I paid for it. His brother needed my car that night? I let him use it, and got into trouble for being late to work because he didn't return it on time.

While I didn't want or need most of the things M brought home, I didn't protest. They had once been part of someone's life, a family heirloom, or useful in some way, and casting them out when they had already been discarded once was something I couldn't do. He didn't work, and rescuing objects and fixing them gave him some kind of purpose. It was a way of caring.

I cleaned out the house many times, trying all my friends' suggestions. My one and only garage sale netted me thirty-two dollars for a week's work and still required driving to Goodwill afterwards. Pickups by various charities were theoretically a win-win but did not account for disgruntled truck drivers who refused to pick up random items because of vague rules no-one told me about. I scheduled a sofa pickup once only to have no-one show up.

The time and effort to clear stuff was daunting but nothing was more of an emotional landmine than the task of sorting: *I choose you, and not you.* For a while I found relief in the Quakers. They took and used everything to furnish homes for new immigrants to America and I drove carloads of stuff across the river to Cambridge where they had their donation center. But they were short-staffed and only opened a few days of the month, and then sporadically, and then never. It was back to hauling stuff to Goodwill and, worse, the town dump.

When the divorce was done, I was left with the house and everything in it–all of it. After a week of carting carloads of stuff to Goodwill and hiring a dumpster, I still had a sizable stash in the basement and attic. But at least that stuff was out of my way and on most days, I could pretend it was gone.

GLP-1 drugs change appetite but that is not the only system affected when body weight shifts. When we lose 15–20% of our body weight, our bodies are being remodeled.

In this chapter we go beyond the question of whether GLP-1 drugs cause muscle loss to the more nuanced question of what happens to muscle when we place the body in sustained, pharmacologic satiety for months or years?

What We Mean by "Muscle"

When people talk about muscle loss, they usually mean one thing when, in reality, there are actually three things to consider.

1. How Much Muscle You Have–This is mass. It's what shows up on a DXA scan as a component of "lean mass."

2. How Good That Muscle Is– This is about muscle quality. Does it contain fat? Is it metabolically active? Is it strong for its size?

3. What That Muscle Can Do–How functional is it? Can you climb stairs? Stand from a chair easily? Carry groceries?

Most GLP-1 trials measure only the first category, lean mass. They show that when people lose significant weight on GLP-1 drugs, roughly one quarter to one third of total weight lost comes from lean mass. This is to be expected as large-scale weight loss almost always includes some lean mass reduction.

Your lean mass percentage can go up while your total muscle mass goes down. If fat drops faster than muscle, you look leaner, even if you have less muscle overall. Appearance and reserve are not the same thing.

Muscle Is a Signaling Organ

Muscle does not grow simply because you eat protein. Signals have to align:

1. Amino acids must rise above a threshold.
2. The energy supply must be sufficient.
3. Mechanical tension must stimulate growth pathways.

At the center of this process is the molecular switch called mTOR. In the first chapter mTOR was introduced as an energy sensor. Here we can think of it as a construction foreman who doesn't respond to constant background noise. He needs clear, strong signals before he lets his team start their job.

The Pulse Principle

When you eat a solid dose of protein:

- Amino acids spike in the blood.

- mTOR activates.

- Muscle protein synthesis rises.

- Then it shuts off again.

Muscle is designed for pulses, not constant drip. If amino acids are mildly elevated all day, the muscle response is weaker. It's like having background noise that you don't pay attention to rather than clear, distinct instructions from your boss. This is sometimes called the "muscle full" effect.

More is not always more because amplitude and energy matter too. If you are in a sustained calorie deficit, the body activates energy-conserving pathways that partially suppress muscle-building signals, even if protein is present. The message is "we have an energy crisis so don't build anything until we can get more energy."

What GLP-1 Therapies Change

GLP-1 drugs change the environment in which muscle operates.

1. Energy Intake Drops

This is the dominant effect. People eat much less. Sustained calorie reduction shifts the body toward using stored fuel such as fat and some lean tissue. Any major weight loss — surgery, diet, or medication — reduces both.

2. Insulin Patterns Change

Insulin becomes more efficient and less chronically elevated which is metabolically beneficial. But muscle building depends partly on insulin's synergy with amino acids. Lower background insulin may reduce baseline anabolic tone.

3. Glucagon Dynamics Differ by Drug

Some GLP-1 drugs suppress glucagon tone. Others (dual and triple agonists) intentionally stimulate glucagon receptors. Glucagon influences how the liver handles amino acids. Depending on the drug class, amino acids may clear more slowly or be oxidized more rapidly. We do not yet have detailed 24-hour amino acid profiling under chronic therapy as this would require long-term human tracer studies, making them hard to do..

4. Stomach Emptying Slows

This is especially so in early treatment. Protein enters the bloodstream more slowly and spikes may flatten. This long term flattening of protein pulses may change metabolic dynamics in the body.

"Just Eat More Protein"

A common response I see doctors giving their patients is to tell them to eat more protein. Higher protein intake during weight loss does help preserve lean mass, but several realities complicate that advice under GLP-1 therapy:

- Meals are smaller.
- Appetite is lower.
- Protein can be harder to tolerate than carbohydrates.
- Energy intake remains suppressed.

If someone consumes enough total protein but never reaches the per-meal threshold required to strongly stimulate mTOR, the anabolic signal may be muted.

We do not have direct studies showing that GLP-1 therapy creates amino-acid resistance. What we do know is that even in optimized weight-loss trials with lifestyle counseling, lean mass declines during GLP-1–mediated weight loss. So while protein intake can attenuate loss, it does not eliminate it. And "just eating more protein" cannot override sustained energy deficit and hence, a strong catabolic (demolition) signal.

"Just Lift Weights"

Resistance training is powerful as it can activate muscle growth pathways independent of insulin. In general weight-loss studies (not involving GLP-1 drugs) show that resistance training preserves muscle. However it rarely builds substantial new muscle in significant calorie deficit.

GLP-1 trials did not include standardized, supervised strength programs. So the lean mass outcomes we see reflect typical real-world exercise patterns, and not optimized mechanical loading. If muscle is not mechanically stimulated during weight loss, some loss is expected. Resistance training is necessary if preservation is the goal but it may not be sufficient on its own when energy remains chronically low.

Ripped vs Robust

Here is where confusion often begins. When the fat just under your skin (called subcutaneous fat) disappears, muscle becomes visible. Shoulders pop, abs are defined, and the body looks more sculpted. One of the most common things people have said to me when they lost weight was, "Look, Dr. Loh, I have more muscle now."

Their DXA reports, however, would show net muscle mass loss. My patients equated being able to see their muscles with having more muscle. They could see the muscle because the overlying fat layer was gone. Someone can look dramatically "fitter" while having lost several pounds of lean mass.

Lean mass percentage tends to rise during GLP-1 therapy while absolute lean mass often falls. Let's look at why this happens.

Lean Mass Percentage vs. Lean Mass — Why the Difference Matters

Here is where numbers can quietly mislead us. Imagine someone who weighs 220 pounds. His body composition is made up of

- 120 pounds in lean mass
- 100 pounds in fat mass

That means lean mass makes up about 55% of their body weight.

Now imagine they lose 40 pounds on a GLP-1 drug and now weigh 180 pounds. Let's say that 30 pounds of that loss was fat and 10 pounds was lean mass.

Now they have:

- 110 pounds of lean mass
- 70 pounds of fat mass

Lean mass now makes up **61%** of their body weight and so the percentage went up. But notice that the **total amount of lean mass went down**. They have less muscle in absolute terms, even though the proportion of their body that is lean is higher.

Why this matters is because when people say, "my lean mass improved," they may mean the percentage improved. Since muscle function depends on how much contractile tissue you actually have and not just what fraction of your body it represents, it means that you've lost strength.

So in short, if you shrink the fat layer faster than the muscle layer, the muscle becomes more visible and can look more defined. But the total muscle reserve is likely lower than before, and this has clinical significance as your risk for frailty goes up..

Regaining Muscle — Is It Likely?

You've probably noticed that when weight is regained after dieting, fat often returns more easily than muscle. This has long been observed in non-drug weight-loss research and is because fat and muscle do not rebuild at the same speed, or under the same rules. After significant weight loss:

- Resting energy expenditure is lower.
- Appetite-regulating hormones often shift in favor of hunger.
- The body becomes metabolically efficient at storing energy.

Fat tissue is biologically designed for rapid energy storage. When calories increase again, adipose (fat) cells can refill quickly. Muscle is different. Rebuilding muscle requires:

- Adequate protein
- Sufficient total energy
- Mechanical loading
- **Time**

Muscle growth is metabolically expensive (costs energy) while fat storage is metabolically efficient. So if someone loses fat and muscle, the body tends to regain fat mass more readily than lean mass. This pattern has been observed in traditional dieting and in some bariatric surgery follow-up studies. Muscle recovery requires deliberate stimulus, whereas fat restoration requires only surplus energy. That asymmetry is biologically sensible and clinically important.

We do not yet have long-term body composition data after extended GLP-1 therapy followed by discontinuation. The question remains open as to whether prolonged pharmacologic satiety shifts the muscle system toward a lower equilibrium that is difficult to reverse. We will return to that question in the chapter on metabolic hysteresis.

Beyond Muscle: The System

Muscle is, of course, part of a larger system that includes bone, tendon, nerves, balance, and energy expenditure. When body mass decreases significantly, bone loading decreases, total energy expenditure decreases, and mechanical strain patterns shift.

Weight loss of any kind — surgical, dietary, pharmacologic — influences these systems. GLP-1 trials were designed to evaluate cardiometabolic outcomes, not evaluate decades-long trajectories of frailty, bone density, or neuromuscular decline.

The musculoskeletal system is integrated and changing one component leads to a domino effect. If muscle mass declines, bone loading changes; if mechanical stimulus declines, connective tissue has to adapt. Bone is a living tissue that strengthens in response to load. Muscles pull on it during walking, lifting, and resistance training, to stimulate bone remodeling. When body weight drops substantially (through surgery, dieting, or medication), the skeleton carries less mechanical load.

In bariatric surgery research and other large weight-loss studies, substantial weight reduction has been associated with increased bone turnover and measurable declines in bone mineral density over time. The bone adapts to the forces placed upon it. Reduce the force, and the stimulus to maintain density declines. Since muscle and bone are partners, if resistance training is not implemented and maintained, both tissues receive a weaker signal to preserve structure.

Some individuals with obesity already have relatively low muscle mass and early bone vulnerability, a pattern sometimes described as osteosarcopenic obesity. In that state, excess fat coexists with reduced structural reserve. When large amounts of fat are removed body weight normalizes but muscle mass may decline even further and bone loading decreases.

A person can move from "osteosarcopenic obesity" to a leaner form that still carries low muscle reserve, sometimes now described as lean sarcopenia (muscle loss), with or without osteopenia (low bone density). The weight looks "healthier" with an "improved" BMI, but the structural reserve may have worsened depending on age, baseline muscle and bone status, rate of weight loss, resistance training, and nutritional sufficiency.

Fat can hide fragility. When the fat layer is reduced, the underlying structural capacity matters more. That is why successful therapy should not be defined by weight reduction alone but by **whether the person is more or less frail at the lighter weight.**

Bottom Line

GLP-1 therapies produce substantial weight loss.

→Most of that loss is fat.

→A measurable portion is lean mass.

In other words, when you lose weight, **you lose both muscle and fat**

When you regain weight, **you mostly regain fat**

Muscle preservation requires:

- Adequate protein in sufficient per-meal doses
- Resistance training with real mechanical load
- Sufficient total energy to support an anabolic response

Lean mass percentage may improve while total muscle mass declines. Just because you can see your muscles does not mean you *have* a lot of muscle. BMI reduction/weight loss does not equal musculoskeletal health.

In individuals with low baseline muscle mass, older adults, or those with early bone loss, → **substantial weight reduction without deliberate muscle protection can shift body composition toward vulnerability rather than resilience.**

****

Chapter 5

When I was in college, my parents and friends would send snacks from home–prawn crackers, haw flakes, dried cuttle-fish, preserved salted prunes, pineapple tarts. I'd look at them now and then and imagine their taste but actually eating them was off limits. They represented home, and I couldn't just obliterate them in my gut.

In the second semester of freshman year I joined some people from my dorm for dinner at a Chinese restaurant. The food was unrecognizable and confusing. There were chicken pieces so thickly battered, they tasted like fried dough. Everyone kept saying how it was such good Chinese food and looked at me brightly, expecting–was it validation?—from me. I had been taught that if I had nothing good to say, I should be silent. At that age my skill in tact depended on putting food in my mouth to accomplish that goal. I tore open the wrapper to the biscuit in front of me and bit into it nervously. It was sweet, and crispy and then strangely chewy and tasteless. *Dude, did you just eat the fortune?* The entire table was staring at me. Then everyone started cracking open their biscuits and showing me their fortunes. *Didn't you know? Aren't you from China? Don't they have fortune cookies there?* My mother had told me that American food was full of fillers but I didn't know they resorted to paper. Who the hell would put paper in a biscuit?

Later, lying in the dark in my apartment while yet another car alarm went off, I felt lost. Even the Chinese food here was foreign. I broke down and unwrapped one Haw Flakes cylinder. Made of dried hawberries pressed into thin discs, I had loved them as a child. I bit into each crisp wafer, savouring its sweetness while feeling guilty for using up my store of–what? It wasn't food, or supplies of any kind. Connection. I was using up my store of connection to my past, to who I was, to how it used to be.

This new world was unfamiliar, mildly menacing in its bluntness, and quite disorienting. Everything I knew to be true was challenged in unexpected ways. While sitting in calculus class I overheard a student behind me ask his friend when the attack on Pearl Harbor was. *April, I think?* was the reply. A wave of panic hit me. Wait, had I been wrong all this while? I resisted the urge to turn around. Pearl Harbor was in America after all; they should know.

It was in December, said another voice, and I relaxed. *December 7th.* I froze. Doubt flooded in. Wasn't it December 8th? My memory had always been solid, but now I couldn't figure out why I was losing it. Later I learned that December 7th in America was December 8th in Asia where I was from. Of course. Even explained, such experiences were destabilizing.

My friends' parents who hoarded did so for a variety of reasons but there is something about the plenitude and abundance of America that sets off a fear of lack and limitations. The more you have the more you fear missing out. When opportunities stretch before you as an unlimited supply, it can be hard to discern excess from enough. Anxiety sets in because we have no stopping rule. Hoarding is blindness to balance, proportion, and flow. The resulting overload is a stunted life, confined and restricted by the allure of more.

Objects become emotionally charged. My biggest accumulations were in books and clothes. Books because they were my proxy parents and mentors. When I needed advice or to learn anything, I turned to books. When I was in need of comfort it was books that provided solace. Books of all kinds–textbooks, self-help, tough love, wisdom, spirituality–were lifelong companions who got me through the darkest periods of my life. To discard such friends would be betrayal.

Clothes were quite the opposite. I bought clothes because I liked fashion. They were ways that I wanted to be seen, and ways to allow parts of me to express. 80% of my wardrobe was untouched. Before America, I had never felt like a geek. In Singapore, the most popular kids were the smartest "all-rounders". In America, intelligence was a liability. My book habit was ingrained from childhood but I started collecting clothes in America. Where books were part of my daily grind, clothes were a kind of vision board, attractive and appealing but rarely lived in. And so my obsessions were grounded in both reality and fantasy as the most entrenched ones are.

Collecting things, and holding on to them, was a way of dealing with a pervasive feeling of inadequacy, of not being enough.

In Chapter 1, we established that immunity is metabolically expensive: cells shift to glycolysis; fever raises energy demand; inflammation reallocates resources. One way that the immune system organizes is through signaling molecules called cytokines. We're used to labeling these molecules 'inflammatory' (hence the term 'inflammatory cytokines') but we should note that they also signal anti-inflammatory measures. One such cytokine is interleukin-6, or IL-6.

During severe infection, IL-6 rises. and GLP-1 rises with it. With GLP-1 drug therapy, IL-6 is also modulated. Why would a hormone used to suppress appetite be woven into inflammatory signaling? Why would a cytokine associated with sickness be capable of stimulating GLP-1 production?

These are not random overlaps. They suggest a shared control system, one that governs energy allocation under stress. Most of what we call "IL-6" in clinical studies is a single number in a lab report. That number does not tell us which cells are signaling, which receptors are engaged, or whether IL-6 is coordinating repair, defense, or metabolic adaptation.

If GLP-1 therapies alter IL-6 tone, we are intervening in a complex communication system that shapes inflammation. To understand the implications, we must first understand how that communication is structured.

IL-6 and IL-1β: More Than "Inflammation"

Like other cytokines, IL-6 is viewed as an inflammatory sign by the medical world. Many studies report "high IL-6" levels as markers of inflammation and the knee-jerk reaction to this is to assume that it is somehow involved in disease progression.

But IL-6 also helps the body decide how to spend energy during a crisis by signaling between muscle, liver, fat, and brain. With the immune system activated, energy demands rise, cells mobilize through metabolic switches that shift how they use fuel, and nutrients are redirected toward defense and repair. IL-6 and other cytokines help coordinate this transition by inducing 'sickness behaviors'. Fever, fatigue, reduced appetite, low mood–these behaviors are part of the body's strategy to conserve energy and mobilize glucose and fatty acids for redirection to the immune army.

The Three "Voices" of IL-6

One reason IL-6 is so difficult to interpret is that it does not signal in only one way. It has at least three distinct signaling modes or three "voices", each capable of producing different outcomes.

1. **A regional voice**
   Countries often form pacts and treaties with each other (e.g. TAC), or they have regional organizations (e.g. ASEAN, The African Union), trade alliances (APEC) or defence agreements (NATO). To coordinate and function, they communicate within themselves. Similarly, in some tissues, IL-6 signals only to specific cell types. In this setting, it often participates in coordinated metabolic responses and acute repair processes.
2. **A global voice**
   When communicating across nations, broader messaging and tone is needed for a particular context. Similarly, IL-6's global voice signals more widely across many tissues. This mode is more commonly associated with sustained inflammatory states and vascular activation.
3. **A local voice**
   This is used to address neighborhood groups, community collectives and local networks. Within the immune system, IL-6 uses this voice. The cytokine can be presented directly from one immune cell to another in adaptive immunity, shaping how T cells develop and respond.

When clinical trials measure IL-6, they don't distinguish which voice is active. They just report a single number in the bloodstream but never tell us which voice IL-6 is using. Is it negotiating energy trades with members of a metabolic axis with its regional voice? Are we sending out a general message to the world? Or is this a committee meeting of the HOA board? Just knowing a number is knowing only that IL-6 is speaking. We have no idea to whom, on what topic, and in what context.

For a clinical trial to give us meaningful information about IL-6, we would need to know which tissues are producing IL-6 (who's talking), which cells are responding (who's listening), and whether IL-6 is participating in repair, defense, or chronic inflammation (the agenda). To date, no clinical trial measuring IL-6 has defined the framework within which it is functioning. This limitation becomes important when we begin to examine how GLP-1 therapies influence immune signaling.

IL-1β: An Upstream Trigger

To be clear, GLP-1 intersects with the immune system through various means. IL-6 plays a prominent role but is not the only actor. Another cytokine, IL-1β, often rises early during inflammatory activation, contributing to fever and helping to initiate the acute phase response. In inflammatory signaling, it is upstream of IL-6 and one of its responsibilities (together with another cytokine, TNF-alpha) is to stimulate IL-6 production. In metabolic disease, IL-1β activity can be elevated. Blocking IL-1 signaling has been shown to improve certain metabolic parameters in specific clinical settings.

GLP-1 receptor activation has been shown in experimental systems to reduce some inflammatory pathways upstream of IL-6, such as IL-1β. In humans, chronic GLP-1 therapy is often associated with lower inflammatory markers. But as with IL-6, a reduced number does not fully describe which immune pathways have been altered. For the rest of this chapter we will focus on IL-6.

Why This Matters for GLP-1

If IL-6 is part of a coordinated energy-allocation system, and if GLP-1 interacts with that system, then changing GLP-1 signaling may alter more than appetite. It may reshape immune–metabolic tone.

Before we can evaluate whether that shift is beneficial, neutral, or context-dependent, we need to understand what IL-6 actually does.

When Inflammation Raises GLP-1

The first hint that GLP-1 and the immune system were linked came not from obesity medicine but from the ICU. Patients there who were severely ill with sepsis, trauma, or other major inflammatory stress, were noted to have increases in their GLP-1 levels. These increases occurred alongside elevations in inflammatory cytokines, including IL-6.

This was unexpected. GLP-1 was seen primarily as a gut hormone that responds to food. Yet during systemic inflammation, when appetite is often reduced, GLP-1 increased even in the absence of normal feeding. Careful human studies using controlled inflammatory challenges showed similar patterns. When inflammation is experimentally induced, cytokines such as IL-6 rise, and GLP-1 levels increase as well.

These observations were associative and did not prove causation, but they raised the question of whether IL-6 could stimulate GLP-1 production. Animal studies provided a mechanistic answer. In experimental models, IL-6 can stimulate intestinal cells to release GLP-1. IL-6 also increases expression of proglucagon, the precursor molecule for GLP-1. When IL-6 signaling is impaired, GLP-1 rise in response to stress is blunted.

In other words, during inflammatory stress, IL-6 can act upstream of GLP-1. This makes physiological sense. In Chapter 1, we described inflammation as an energy-reallocation program. During infection or stress, the body suppresses appetite, mobilizes fuel, and redirects energy toward defense. GLP-1 contributes to appetite suppression and glucose regulation. IL-6 may help initiate that response as part of energy-saving 'sickness behaviors'. GLP-1, in this context, appears not as an isolated satiety hormone but as **part of a coordinated immune–metabolic adaptation**.

When GLP-1 Signals Back Through IL-6

The relationship isn't only unidirectional. IL-6 stimulates GLP-1, and experimental studies have shown that GLP-1 activation can increase IL-6 expression in certain tissues, particularly in fat. In 2022 a paper by Gutierrez et al made this link explicit.

Fat tissue can have different characteristics. Most of the fat we carry is known as white fat and functions somewhat like a portable refrigerator. Fuel (food) can be brought into the refrigerator for storage or moved out and used for energy in different parts of the body like the muscles, heart, liver and kidneys. Brown fat is more like a woodstove. The fuel in it is used to generate heat.

Under some conditions such as cold exposure and severe inflammation, certain populations of white fat known as beige fat can be converted to brown fat. When this happens and the brown fat volume increases, the body burns more energy to make heat. For someone trying to lose weight, this might seem like a good thing because we're wasting more calories even at rest. This is akin to turning the heat up while opening the windows and doors in the winter. While this might give a small advantage towards weight loss, it doesn't usually contribute meaningful caloric deficits. The fire can also get out of control and start consuming other energy stores in the body, including muscles and tissues. That process is called cachexia and can be seen in wasting conditions such as cancer.

In the Gutierrez paper, the group used rodent models to show that GLP-1 signaling stimulates white/beige fat conversion to heat-producing brown fat, a process called 'browning' or thermogenesis (literally, *heat-making*). Other research groups have since confirmed this GLP-1 action. In these studies, IL-6 was required for the full thermogenic response. When IL-6 signaling was blocked or absent, GLP-1-induced browning of white fat was significantly reduced. This establishes a clear mechanistic link in experimental systems: GLP-1 receptor activation → increased IL-6 signaling → activation of thermogenic genes.

In humans using GLP-1 receptor agonists for obesity, **the primary driver of weight loss is reduced food intake**. Energy expenditure changes, including thermogenesis, are modest. While thermogenic pathways are biologically interesting, they do not account for the majority of clinical weight reduction with GLP-1. Reduced intake, and not fat browning, explains most of the weight loss observed in large trials.

Thermogenesis in the Wrong Context

While it sounds like a good idea to burn more calories using thermogenesis, it may actually backfire in certain scenarios. In chronic illnesses such as advanced cancer, heart failure, liver failure, severe pulmonary disease, and chronic kidney disease, patients can develop cachexia from reduced appetite, elevated energy use, and progressive loss of lean mass. In these conditions, inappropriate activation of thermogenic pathways through fat browning has been shown to contribute to energy wasting.

IL-6 is often elevated in cachexia and participates in metabolic dysregulation in that setting. As GLP-1 receptor agonists are increasingly used beyond obesity (including in cardiac populations) it becomes important to ask whether immune–metabolic pathways that are adaptive in obesity might behave differently in individuals already at risk for wasting.

Shared Neural Circuits: Appetite and Immune Signaling

GLP-1 receptors are present in brain regions that regulate appetite and nausea. Activation of these receptors reduces food intake. Cytokines such as IL-6 also influence feeding centers in the brain during infection, contributing to sickness behavior.

GLP-1 does not reproduce the full inflammatory program of illness. However, the neural circuits overlap. Both systems can reduce appetite to influence energy allocation, and interact with hypothalamic pathways in the brain. This convergence reinforces the broader theme that GLP-1 signaling intersects with immune biology. To understand what chronic GLP-1 therapy does to inflammatory tone, we must now distinguish between short-term and long-term immune effects.

Short-Term Signals and Long-Term Tone

If IL-6 can stimulate GLP-1 during inflammation, and GLP-1 can signal through IL-6 in fat tissue, this leads to the next question: What happens to IL-6 when GLP-1 drugs are used chronically? To answer that, we must separate short-term signaling from long-term immune tone.

Acute Effects: What Happens Early?

In experimental systems, GLP-1 receptor activation can transiently engage IL-6–dependent pathways. In the work by Gutiérrez and colleagues, GLP-1 receptor agonism increased IL-6 expression in fat tissue and required IL-6 signaling to induce thermogenic gene programs. In these rodent models, IL-6 was not just incidental but mechanistically necessary for browning.

Other preclinical studies have shown tissue-specific increases in IL-6 signaling shortly after GLP-1 receptor activation. Human data on immediate cytokine changes are far more limited. Most large clinical trials measure inflammatory markers weeks to months after therapy begins. There are few detailed human time-course studies measuring IL-6 in the first hours or days after GLP-1 administration.

Chronic Effects: What Happens Over Time?

Across multiple human trials of GLP-1 receptor agonists in both obesity and type 2 diabetes, inflammatory markers tend to decline over time. Reductions in C-reactive protein (CRP, an inflammatory marker) are consistent findings. Several studies also report decreases in circulating IL-6 concentrations after months of therapy.

These are human data but interpretation requires restraint. Clinical trials measure total circulating IL-6. They do not distinguish between the different "voices" of IL-6, which tissues are involved, or whether immune tone and capacity are being altered differently.

A lower IL-6 value in the bloodstream does not automatically mean that all IL-6–dependent functions have been uniformly suppressed. It just shows a shift in systemic inflammatory markers. Whether that shift represents selective dampening of chronic inflammatory signaling, a broader recalibration of immune tone, or both, is still unknown.

The Interpretive Problem

At this point, three conclusions are well supported:

1. IL-6 can stimulate native GLP-1 production during inflammatory stress (demonstrated in animal models with supportive human associations).
2. GLP-1 receptor activation can engage IL-6–dependent pathways in browning (as demonstrated by Gutiérrez et al. and related experimental work).
3. Chronic GLP-1 therapy in humans is associated with lower circulating inflammatory numbers.

What we do not yet know is equally important:

- Does chronic GLP-1 therapy just reduce the "bad" inflammatory IL-6 functions while preserving its "good" regenerative and repair functions?

- Does lowering baseline inflammation allow us to still mount a strong immune response when needed?

- How does it alter the immune environment differently in fat tissue, muscle, liver, and brain?

Current clinical assays cannot answer these questions. That limitation is important because if IL-6 participates in coordinating energy allocation, tissue repair, and adaptive immunity, then changing its tone is not a trivial intervention. We're not just talking about an intervention involving the local community garden. We're implementing a global initiative that affects the earth's geology. That is a systems biology change that will impact every aspect of our lives.

"Inflammation" and "Anti-Inflammatory" Are Not Yin-Yang

We tend to see inflammation as a villain. If a therapy lowers CRP, that's good. If IL-6 decreases, that's reassuring. Let's clear the body of "inflammation" and we should all live healthily ever after. The logic feels intuitive, but it depends on a simplified (almost to the point of being simplistic) view of the immune system.

The immune system is not a switch with two positions — on/off, inflamed/not inflamed. It is a regulatory network that must constantly make decisions:

- What is dangerous?
- What is harmless?
- Who do we eliminate?
- Who do we tolerate?
- What must be repaired?

Our immune system has to attack pathogens, tolerate commensal gut bacteria, and allow for pregnancy (technically a state where there is a "foreign body" present). It has to repair tissue after injury and balance tumor surveillance with prevention of autoimmunity. Inflammation and anti-inflammation should not be seen as representative of health and disease. One isn't "good" while the other is "bad". More accurately, they are **coordinated phases** within the immune system.

IL-6 itself demonstrates this complexity. In some contexts, IL-6 participates in acute phase responses to stress/inflammation and metabolic adaptation. In others, it contributes to sustained vascular inflammation. In still others, it supports tissue repair and immune differentiation. When GLP-1 receptor agonist trials report lower IL-6 levels, they are reporting a shift in a circulating marker. They are not reporting a full map of immune signaling. A reduced IL-6 value does not tell us:

- Whether regenerative signaling was preserved

- Whether trans-signaling was selectively reduced
- Whether tissue-specific responses were altered differently
- Whether immune burst capacity remains intact

We just know that a number, a marker level, decreased. This is about as exciting and useful as looking out of a building in Times Square and reporting that there are 631 people in the area. What are they doing? Are they in a parade? Are they protesting? Participating in a dance flash mob? Or are they mostly taking selfies, window-shopping, and buying discounted theater tickets? 631 people could be doing very different activities which affect the environment, safety, noise levels, and traffic.

As GLP-1 drug use expands beyond obesity and diabetes into cardiac, renal, and other chronic conditions, the framing of these drugs as broadly "anti-inflammatory" may create a sense of conceptual closure, as if lowering inflammatory markers is self-evidently beneficial across all contexts. But immune modulation is never context-free.

In some diseases, reducing chronic inflammatory tone may be advantageous while in others, immune signaling may be required for repair. Yet others may need a tight balance between energy conservation and immune activation. The immune system operates across gradients, tissues, and time scales. Just as military forces can attack and defend in one part of the world, and conduct peace-keeping tasks in another, the immune system is capable of simultaneous attack and tolerance in different compartments of the body.

To evaluate GLP-1 receptor agonists responsibly, we must move beyond the reductionist good-versus-bad framing of cytokines. Our task as clinicians and scientists is not to accept "anti-inflammatory" as a static goal. We need to ask which pathways were altered and when, what tissues were involved, and what the downstream consequences are.

Medicine today operates within a framework in which pharmaceutical trials heavily shape clinical understanding. The trials are designed with specific endpoints. Importantly, **they measure only what they are powered to**

measure. If something is not measured, it is not mentioned or accounted for. Medical organizations rely on published endpoints and "guidelines" and then incorporate those into "standards of care". We need to pause and take in the uncomfortable fact that such "standards of care" rely on guideline-based algorithms and not outcomes for our patients. If we are not careful, we begin to equate what was measured with what is known and forget to ask what was not measured, and why.

Understanding the immune–metabolic architecture of GLP-1 does not invalidate clinical trial results. But it reminds us that a biomarker shift is not the same as a systems-level map. What is called for is not cynicism but disciplined curiosity followed by rigorous thinking and questioning.

Bottom Line

GLP-1 signaling sits inside a larger immune–metabolic control system.

Cytokines such as IL-6 can stimulate GLP-1 during inflammatory stress, and GLP-1 signaling can in turn engage IL-6–dependent pathways in tissues such as fat.

While chronic GLP-1 therapy often lowers circulating inflammatory markers, those numbers do not reveal how immune signaling has been reshaped across tissues or functions.

****

Chapter 6

I've fallen into the trap before: You have too much stuff, so you go to the store and buy more stuff in the form of bins and boxes and linen-lined baskets. It feels virtuous, and satisfying because soon, the house will be organized, and pretty. It will have the smell of scented candles and cedar blocks for the closet. The spice jars will be labeled and all shoes will be nested in a compact shoe cabinet with cedar shoe trees snuggled in each one.

In other words, our solution for too much is *even more*. There's nuance though, because it's more of the "right stuff"–folders and binders and hampers and carts–all in the name of giving everything a home. Storage hacking is the way we handle excess. If your clothes don't fit you can double your closet size with tiered hangers. If your towels are spilling out, you need towel ladders, extra hooks, and towel bars. Let's maximize your kitchen cabinets with tiered dish holders and pull-out racks. And while we're at it you should get that egg organizer for the fridge, because the eggs look better in them than in the carton.

What we won't acknowledge is that we're afraid to let go. Things that got us where we are today, things that defined us–what will happen when they go? Who are we without the stuff?

My office was covered in papers, and my room with clothes. I bought things because I couldn't find the ones I had. If I let go of letters and cards, the pens I brought home from the hospital, the stress-reliever squish toy from the physician's burnout prevention committee, the volumes of board-review MKSAP booklets, the thirteen pairs of trauma scissors (they really are very useful), and the many pairs of hospital socks with grippers on the soles–if I let go of them, I might need them one day. I might lose touch with who I am, and I might have to fill the space with some new kind of meaning. Or I might discover that the object was never as necessary as the identity it protected, and I would have to relearn how to move in the void.

———————————————————————

We tend to think of molecules in simple categories: Cholesterol is "bad", inflammation is "bad", and cytokines are "inflammatory." IL-6 is often placed in that last category because...it rises in obesity, it rises in diabetes, and in vascular disease. When doctors see it fall, they often interpret that as improvement. They treat it like a toxin when it is, in fact, a messenger.

And like most messengers in biology, what it says depends on context. Sometimes IL-6 rises sharply and briefly, for example, during exercise, during infection, and after injury. In those moments, it helps redirect energy, mobilize fuel, and coordinate repair. At other times, IL-6 stays modestly elevated for months or years, as in chronic metabolic disease. In that setting, it can contribute to vascular dysfunction and long-term damage. The difference is not simply how much IL-6 is present but also timing.

A brief signal can help adaptation while a chronic signal can erode resilience. Before deciding that less IL-6 is always better, we have to understand what the signal is doing in each situation.

What GLP-1 Therapy Does — and Does Not — Show About IL-6

GLP-1 drugs are often described as "anti-inflammatory." In many long-term studies, people taking these medications show modest reductions in inflammatory markers like IL-6 and C-reactive protein. That is encouraging, especially to individuals with chronic low-grade inflammation linked to obesity and diabetes, but those reductions come with important caveats.

First, most trials measure IL-6 in a single fasting blood sample. They do not measure how IL-6 behaves during stress, exercise, injury, or infection. We do not know what "voice" IL-6 is speaking with. Second, many of the observed reductions in IL-6 may reflect weight loss and improved metabolic health rather than a direct immune effect of the drug. If you just dieted and lost weight on your own, you would likely have a similar lowering of your IL-6 levels. Third, we do not yet know how GLP-1 therapy affects IL-6 inside specific tissues such as muscle, brain, or eye where timing and local signaling matter more than a blood level.

In other words, we know that chronic GLP-1 therapy can lower systemic inflammatory tone. We are not yet aware of how it reshapes the deeper immune-metabolic choreography that IL-6 participates in. That question becomes more interesting when we look at specific organs.

Muscle: When IL-6 Is a Training Signal

When you exercise, especially for a sustained period, your muscles release IL-6 in large, temporary bursts. That pulse of IL-6 helps release stored energy from the liver and fat tissue, improve insulin sensitivity afterward, and trigger anti-inflammatory signals that help resolve the stress of exercise.

IL-6 also plays a role in muscle repair and adaptation. Studies have shown that appropriate IL-6 signaling helps activate the cells responsible for muscle remodeling. Here again, timing matters. A brief IL-6 spike during exercise can help muscles adapt. A chronically elevated level as in severe illness or cachexia (accelerated muscle loss) can contribute to muscle breakdown.

Now consider GLP-1 therapy. These medications reduce appetite and caloric intake as well as total body mass, including some lean mass. Early in treatment, people sometimes feel fatigued or nauseated, which might make them less active. What we do not know is whether long-term GLP-1 therapy changes how muscle uses IL-6 during training and repair. Does it alter the size of those exercise-induced pulses? Does it affect recovery in older adults at risk of muscle loss? What about people who are losing significant weight (and therefore also losing more muscle)?

While there is no evidence that GLP-1 drugs impair muscle adaptation, there is also no detailed mapping of how muscle-specific IL-6 signaling behaves under chronic metabolic modulation. When millions of people are asked to take a drug for years, those questions deserve to be asked.

The Developing Brain: A System Still Under Construction

GLP-1 drugs are increasingly used in children and young adults. Brain development does not stop in childhood. Synaptic pruning, white matter maturation, and refinement of executive circuits continue through adolescence and into the twenties.

Microglia (the immune cells of the brain) help shape which neural connections are strengthened and which are eliminated. Cytokines, including IL-6, participate in that process. In animal models, altering IL-6 signaling during critical developmental windows can change brain structure and long-term behavior. Too much signaling can disrupt development. Too little can also alter normal trajectories.

Biology rarely works by simple opposites such as "inflammation bad, anti-inflammation good." Signals that we associate with stress or damage often play important roles in normal development. A recent animal study illustrates this point. When healthy male mice were given sustained antioxidant supplementation with N-acetylcysteine and selenium before conception, their offspring developed subtle craniofacial abnormalities. The finding does not mean antioxidants are dangerous in general. Rather, it reminds us that systems built around signaling—whether redox molecules or cytokines—operate within a balanced range. Pushing a signal persistently in one direction can disturb developmental programs that depend on precise timing and dose. IL-6 belongs to this same category. Often labeled simply as an inflammatory cytokine, in the developing brain its signals help guide normal neural growth and organization. The question is not whether a signal is good or bad, but how it is being used by the system.

GLP-1 receptor agonists are now approved for adolescents with obesity. Short-term trials show weight loss and acceptable safety profiles. What we do not have are multi-decade studies of individuals who begin therapy during adolescence and continue long-term. Again, there is no current evidence that GLP-1 therapy harms brain development but also no evidence mapping how chronic metabolic and immune recalibration interacts with a brain that is still refining its circuitry.

Stroke and Brain Injury: Early Harm, Later Repair

After a stroke or traumatic brain injury, IL-6 levels rise quickly. Higher early IL-6 levels are associated with more severe injury and worse short-term outcomes. In the acute stage, IL-6 participates in the inflammatory cascade that can expand damage.

As the brain transitions from injury to repair, IL-6 signaling also becomes involved in activating supportive glial cells, promoting new blood vessel formation, and supporting neuronal survival pathways. Research shows that removing IL-6 entirely can hinder aspects of recovery. So the signal that is associated with early injury severity also participates in later remodeling and repair.

GLP-1 drugs are being studied for potential neuroprotective effects and may reduce stroke risk in people with diabetes. What we do not know is how chronic GLP-1 therapy interacts with the time-structured immune response that unfolds after brain injury. Does it dampen harmful excess? Does it alter repair, or do both? We do not yet have those answers.

Alzheimer's Disease: Protection and Pathology in the Same Molecule

In Alzheimer's Disease, IL-6 levels are often elevated in the brain and in the bloodstream. Chronic inflammation is part of the disease landscape, but early in the disease process, immune activation is not purely destructive. Microglia, the brain's immune cells, attempt to clear toxic amyloid deposits and maintain neuronal health. Cytokines, including IL-6, participate in that early *protective* response.

Over time however, sustained inflammatory signaling can contribute to synaptic loss and neurodegeneration. The same molecule can participate in early protection and later pathology. GLP-1 drugs are being investigated as potential therapies in neurodegenerative disease, in part because of their metabolic and anti-inflammatory effects. What remains unclear is how long-term shifts in immune tone affect a disease measured over decades.

Flattening inflammation may help in some stages and may be neutral or damaging in others.

The Eye: Ischemia in a Confined Space

The optic nerve head is where the optic nerve leaves and blood vessels enter the eye. If it swells and compresses on the blood vessels, blood flow to the eye is suddenly reduced, leading to injury. This condition is called non-arteritic anterior ischemic optic neuropathy or (thank goodness!) NAION (pronounced "nay-on").

Research shows that after blood flow to the eye drops, inflammatory signals rise, including IL-6. High IL-6 contributes to the inflammatory response that can worsen edema. However it also activates survival pathways in retinal ganglion cells in the eye and may support nerve recovery in certain contexts. In chronic inflammatory eye diseases, blocking IL-6 can reduce damage while with acute injury, some IL-6 signaling may be part of the repair attempt.

Recently, observational studies have reported an association between GLP-1 receptor agonist use and NAION. These findings do not definitively establish causation, but it is worthwhile to note that bariatric surgery patients have the same risk factors, lose more weight, and are subject to the same labile blood pressure conditions that seem to precipitate NAION. Yet, over years of bariatric surgery data, this has not been a concern associated with those patients.

What is clear is that IL-6 participates in the entire arc of optic nerve injury, from inflammation to attempted repair. How chronic metabolic therapy intersects with that arc remains an open question.

Vaccines: Educating Immune System

We often think of vaccination as "making antibodies". A better way to see it is as a way of instructing the immune system.

IL-6 uses its "local voice" to talk to cells within the immune community. It activates the dendritic cells which present antigens to T cells and teaches them how to respond. It also helps support the formation of germinal centers in lymph nodes where B cells refine their antibodies. Once the B-cells start producing antibodies, they are called plasma cells, and their survival is sustained by IL-6 action. Blocking IL-6 signaling in other clinical contexts can modestly blunt vaccine responses.

We do not know whether GLP-1 drugs meaningfully alter vaccine responses. No large trials have directly tested this. People with obesity and diabetes already have variable vaccine responses. Improving metabolic health may help, and altering immune tone may also have effects. The point is not that GLP-1 therapy impairs immunity but that cytokines like IL-6 are part of how immune memory is built. When a therapy recalibrates immune tone for years, it is reasonable to ask how that recalibration interacts with immune education.

What This Chapter Ultimately Asks

Across muscle, brain development, stroke, Alzheimer's disease, optic nerve injury, and vaccination, we see a pattern: IL-6 is not a single-purpose inflammatory molecule but a context-dependent coordinator. It can contribute to harm, support adaptation and repair, or do both at different times in the same tissue.

GLP-1 receptor agonists clearly improve metabolic health for many patients. But when we chronically modulate a system that coordinates energy, immunity, and repair, we are not just adjusting one dial. We are reshaping a network. Before declaring that less IL-6 is universally better, we should understand what functions depend on its proper timing.

Bottom Line

IL-6 is not simply an inflammatory to be lowered across the board but a timing-sensitive coordinator that helps the body allocate energy, repair tissue, refine the developing brain, respond to injury, and build immune memory.

GLP-1 receptor agonists clearly improve metabolic health for many people. But when we use a long-term therapy that reshapes metabolic and immune tone, we are not just reducing a lab value but also recalibrating a network.

We do not yet fully understand the downstream consequences of chronically modulating a molecule that plays different roles at different stages of life and disease.

****

Chapter 7

Picture me walking, almost running, but not quite. From afar I might look purposeful, determined – driven even. The truth is, I am *paced.*

I'm a sophomore in college, and there's a song running in my head. The guitar bass line is steady, brisk, no-nonsense. The first time I heard that bass was in a Johnny Cash song. *Folsom Prison Blues* and that bass like the train that's taunting me–get out, get out, get out.

This song is different but its impulse, its lineage is unmistakable. That train is still there, egging me–keep up, get going, *move it*–and it's to that musical chugging that I'm power walking to.

Freshman year hadn't delivered. I was friendless, bored, and scared of *coasting.* I was angry. It might have been good advice: just take the easy courses for the grades and make that med school application look great. But that would mean four years of not learning anything, and draining my family's money for nothing. I couldn't do that kind of time, and the song that suddenly came up in the bookstore seemed like a message from the Wise Ones in the middle of a quest: *move.*

I am walking to my biology advisor. I am walking to meet a professor. I am walking because if I don't I will end up stuck in a rut. It might be great for med school but it would mean I'd never get to live life on my terms. I don't know the lyrics of the song–something about Elvis–*Graceland, Memphis, Tennessee.* No matter, because there's only the relentless drone of the guitar in my head, the surreal lick twanging above it and I keep walking.

The biology advisor will approve all graduate level classes and independent study for me, and the meeting with the professor will get me the signature I need to declare a second major in classical languages and literature. In all this, I will meet people I'll come to love and trust. My whole life is about to change and I am on the brink of becoming who I am now but it doesn't matter.

Do it, move it, shove it, make it–that's what the song is saying. And me–I'm just walking.

***

I don't even remember his name but I guess I was heartbroken, and I needed to move. It was my first year in medical school and my memories are compressed so tightly they have lost distinction. But there is a very faint image of moving into my own basement studio apartment in Brookline. The door. Me, writing. A single word, a piece of paper, stuck to the door as if to baptize my new home: Graceland.

I had fifty boxes of books, four ceiling height bookcases and two waist high ones. I didn't really know anyone in med school. Many of my classmates were SMEDS (six-year meds) who had known each other for two years prior to med school. I was in a different early acceptance program and there were only a handful of us. We got together once, for a photograph for the department, an uninspiring and forgettable moment. But somehow, somewhere, Ed, a SMED, heard about my move and asked if he could help.

That's how he ended up staring in shock at my fifty boxes of books in the middle of a Boston winter. *You read all of them?* he asked. I felt bad. They looked even heavier now that we actually had to move them. But he was too much of a gentleman to let me lift anything so my part in the 'we' was hovering guiltily beside him as he carried each box to his car. (We were in medical school, so doing something practical like using a dolly was just too smart for us!).

We made several trips and each time, I played Paul Simon's Graceland album. When I like something I get obsessive. I can loop a song for ten hours, re-watch a favourite program, re-read a poem over and over and find something new each time. Ed never complained, just moved boxes and listened–to the music, to me crying, to my sombre silence.

I unpacked the boxes that first weekend in my new apartment, filling the air with lyrics that spoke of hope, possibility, and redemption, letting the song imprint itself in the continuing story of me.

***

The house had never been what I envisioned. It was a fixer-upper whose fixes required more fixing, since M heavily improvised on them himself. We lived in an eternal construction zone made more hazardous by the stuff M brought in. It never reached full hoarder status but it was cluttered and uninviting and left me feeling ashamed.

Once, my mother visited and asked, "How did this happen? You were always so fastidious about your room." It happened from overwhelm, and constant struggle. My life with M wasn't working out but I could not fail. It was up to me to get my relationship to an A, up to me to keep the place organized, up to me to make things work. Deep down I had really given up but my self-expectations did not let up and that misalignment grated on me.

When M finally moved out, I had my chance. Re-energized, I started sorting out my things from whatever he had left behind. I put them in trashbags with tags for clothes, shoes, widgets, and brought them to the aptly named Goodwill. The biggest blessing of my house was the light. Even in the coldest winter, crisp sunlight poured through the living room and kitchen. The night I finally emptied out the living room, I lay down on the warped wood floors, listening as candlelight danced with their reflection in the windows. I'd lived nineteen years like a human trampoline, *falling, flying, or tumbling in turmoil* and I'd finally bounced off.

Losing love is like a window in your heart

Everybody sees you're blown apart,

Everybody sees the wind blow

There's no obligations now. And so at last, I could rest.

***

It took three years after Tom's death to go through his stuff. And when I did, making decisions on what to do with it was too much. I made piles, bought plastic bins and stuffed them away. And then I medicated with work.

By the time my dog Tula died, it was grief upon years of unprocessed grief. She had been by my side for sixteen years, even on the day we made the decision to disconnect life support for Tom. She was there in the ICU hidden in the bag I carried when he took his last breath. She was there waiting patiently as I lay beside his body to say goodbye. She was there that night when the sky turned green from the rare sight of the Northern Lights, and when I went back to work the next day.

And the many deaths wedged in between life, derailing dreams and schedules, upending new starts–those who want to live forever don't realize that the longer you live the more you'll lose. The uncles with liver cancer, childhood pets, the classmate who drowned, the one who had a high fever one day and slipped into a coma, and whose parents couldn't look you in the eye at the crematorium because you grew up together and you're still here, the shriveled grandparents, the people you trained with and signed out patients to, the Attending who no-one visited in the nursing home, and the one who died in the middle of a tennis game swinging at life with his last—

The losses keep growing, all building up to the ultimate loss in our own deaths, but by that time we're ready because there's no-one left to live for. Here are tufts of Tula's hair caught in the tiny bows she wore. Here is her smell on her bed, and here are the oxtail bones she buried under her pillows. Tula was a witness to so many of those losses and losing her was like losing a whole life.

I'm walking because it was our routine, but I can't face the memories of our usual path, and so I'm striking out in a new direction, a new walk. This song that we listened to for weeks when M moved out, it's come back the same and different. This time I'm walking with *ghosts and empties*, this time with the broken window of the heart, *everybody* ***feels*** *the wind blow*. Where we are is not where we began. It is the Second Law.

Imagine jumping on a trampoline. *Boing, boing, boing.* When you get off, the trampoline looks the same. No-one can even tell that you were on it a minute ago.

Now imagine it's a beach day and you jump onto wet sand as you play at the water's edge. The sand compresses with your weight. Even after you move from that spot you'll leave evidence behind in your footprints.

Same force, same person, two very different materials. One rebounds cleanly while the other carries a memory of the impact. That difference is the essence of **metabolic hysteresis**.

In a system without hysteresis, changes are reversible while changes within a hysteretic system leave structural traces. Weight regulation in the human body behaves much more like jumping on wet sand than a trampoline.

The Myth of Perfect Reversibility

We are often told that weight loss is simple. Just eat less, lose weight, and then you can eat "normally" again and maintain that weight. In my practice I ran an intensive three-month long weight loss program that used meal replacements and focused on nutrition, movement, sleep, and behavior change. Patients lost anywhere from forty to sixty pounds in twelve weeks, achieving surgical results without the surgery.

After the twelve weeks, almost everyone asked when they could "go back to eating their old way". *Never*, I told them, *not unless you want your old weight back*. They seemed genuinely surprised at this. It was unreasonable, or extreme, they said, to only eat fresh produce and avoid junk foods and dessert as a way of life. Couldn't they at least take a break every now and then and eat some of their old favorites?

But biology does not bargain. When someone gains weight over years, the body adapts to that higher weight. Appetite recalibrates, energy expenditure shifts, fat cells enlarge and sometimes increase in number, and hormone sensitivity falls. When weight is then lost — whether through dieting, surgery, or medication — the body does not simply return to its original pre-weight-gain state. It carries memory. **The same body weight after weight loss is not biologically identical to that weight before weight gain**. That is what we call metabolic hysteresis.

A Practical Example

Consider a person who weighed 90 kg, gained to 110 kg, and then lost back to 90 kg. On the scale, they are "back where they started" but physiologically:

- Their resting metabolic rate may be lower than it was the first time they weighed 90 kg.

- Their hunger signals may be stronger.

- Their body may defend fat mass more aggressively.

- Their muscle mass may be lower and fat percentage higher than before.

- The number on the scale matches while the biology does not.

Why This Matters

If the body behaved like a trampoline, weight loss would be straightforward and stable. But the body is more like wet sand, and so weight loss changes the structure of the system. Weight regain follows predictable biological pressures, and each lose-regain cycle may subtly reshape our physiologic terrain.

This isn't to say weight loss is futile. It means weight loss is not mechanically reversible. Understanding this changes how we think about dieting, medication, long-term therapy, and stopping therapy. And this, of course, changes what we should measure.

What Actually Changes in the Body

If metabolic hysteresis is the "footprint in the sand," what exactly is being imprinted? The body changes during weight gain and weight loss, and some of those changes do not fully reverse.

1. Your Metabolism Slows More Than You Expect

When people lose weight, their metabolism drops, which makes sense. Smaller bodies burn fewer calories. Yet research shows that after significant weight loss, the body often burns fewer calories than would be predicted based on its new size alone. In other words, metabolism becomes more efficient ("thriftier") than expected. Even years later, some individuals who have lost substantial weight still burn fewer calories than someone of the same size who has never dieted.

That means the same calorie intake that once maintained weight may now cause regain. This is a measurable biological adaptation.

2. The Brain Recalibrates Hunger

Weight gain changes how the brain responds to food signals. Areas that regulate hunger, satiety, and reward adjust to higher levels of body fat and circulating hormones. When weight is lost later, hunger signals often increase, food becomes more attention-grabbing, and the body perceives the new lower weight as a deficit state.

Even if the scale reads "normal," the brain may still be operating as though weight needs to be restored. This helps explain why maintaining weight loss can feel harder than losing weight in the first place. The control system has shifted.

3. Fat and Muscle Do Not Change Symmetrically

Your weight is made up of fat, muscle, bone, water, and connective tissue. During weight loss, a portion of the loss comes from muscle. The proportion varies, but muscle loss *is* common. With weight regain, a larger proportion of regained weight tends to be fat. Muscle recovery often lags behind fat recovery and in the older, more anabolic resistance person, muscle may never recover.

The result? A person can return to the same body weight but with higher body fat percentage, lower muscle mass, and lower resting metabolic rate. Simply put, when you lose weight, you're losing both fat and muscle.When you gain weight, it's mostly fat you're regaining. The number may be the same but the body composition tells a different story.

Fat Tissue Itself Changes

Fat cells enlarge during weight gain, and, in some cases, new fat cells are formed. After weight loss fat cells shrink in size but the total number of fat cells does not decrease. That means that the body retains the structural capacity to store fat efficiently. In addition, fat tissue undergoes changes in immune activity and cellular signaling during obesity. While some of this improves with weight loss, not all of it fully resets. The terrain has been reshaped.

Putting It Together

Weight gain alters metabolic rate, brain signaling. fat tissue structure, and muscle mass. Weight loss changes those variables again but they do not trace back along the same path. Instead of returning to its original shape like a trampoline, the system retains impressions like wet sand. That is why weight regain is so common. Your body is shaped by its history; it remembers.

Why Weight Regain Is Predictable

Once we understand that the body behaves like wet sand and not a trampoline, the next question becomes why weight regain happens so often.

1. The Calorie Equation Changes After Weight Loss

Many people were taught that if you reduce calories by a certain amount, you lose a predictable amount of weight. That assumes metabolism stays constant, but it doesn't. As weight drops, the body requires fewer calories to function. Muscles burn fewer calories, daily movement often decreases subconsciously, and hormonal signals adjust. As we saw in chapter 1, our energy requirement equations are approximations and some physiologic adjustments (such as lowered energy needs from lowered inflammation) are like money-laundering in that they are often hard to account for completely.

The energy deficit that produced weight loss at the beginning becomes smaller over time. And once weight stabilizes at a lower level, the number of calories required to maintain that lower weight is often less than what would have maintained that same weight before weight gain ever occurred.

That means returning to previous eating patterns, even if moderate, may now create a positive energy balance. The body is now operating under new rules.

2. Muscle and Fat Do Not Return the Same Way

We've already seen this: when losing weight, you tend to lose both fat and muscle. When you gain the weight back, you mostly regain fat. This matters because muscle is more metabolically active than fat. Simply put, this means it burns more calories at rest than fat. If someone regains fat but little or no muscle, then their metabolism is lower than it was the first time they weighed that amount. Their body composition has shifted, even if their weight number has not, and this sets them up for future regain. The sand has been reshaped.

3. The Body Defends Against Weight Loss

After weight loss, hunger signals often increase. Food may seem more appealing as satiety feels less durable. This is part of the body's regulatory system trying to restore what it interprets as lost reserves.

When weight regain occurs, the system often stabilizes at a new point. That new point however, may differ in composition and metabolic efficiency from where the person began. That loop — down in weight, up again, **but not along the same path** — is metabolic hysteresis in action. While this is seen in all forms of weight loss, weight regain after stopping GLP-1 drugs is faster than regain from stopping lifestyle-only weight loss because the 'locked in' signal they impose is so strong. These drugs profoundly alter metabolic and immune physiology in ways we are still far from understanding.

GLP-1 Medications in a Hysteretic System

GLP-1 medications strongly reduce appetite, slow stomach emptying, and alter brain responses to food. They act like an external force pressing on the body to force a change in energetics. In our analogy, it's like pressing someone deeper into the sand.

During treatment, food intake decreases and blood sugar improves. Over time, weight drops and cardiometabolic markers often improve. These effects can be profound and beneficial but underneath, the body is still adapting. The drug overrides hunger-regulating circuits, suppressing them. Metabolism decreases with weight as muscle mass declines. Mechanical loading on bone changes.

When the drug is discontinued, appetite signals return. Energy expenditure remains lower due to prior weight loss and our evolutionary bias towards storing fat resumes. Clinical studies show that 60-70% of lost weight is often regained within a year after stopping therapy. By 18-24 months, we see a near return to baseline weight, although fat weight is now higher. This is not surprising if we remember the wet sand. We jumped onto it, pressing it down. And when we walked away, it was not the same as before.

Questions to Discuss With Your Doctor

If weight regulation behaves like wet sand rather than a trampoline, then starting or stopping a GLP-1 medication is not a trivial decision. We are talking about a meaningful intervention in a system that remembers.

Here are questions worth discussing openly with your physician.

1. What Is the Real Goal of This Treatment?

    - Is the primary goal weight reduction?

    - Is it blood sugar control?

    - Is it cardiovascular risk reduction?

    - Is this expected to be short-term or long-term therapy?

    - Understanding the goal helps clarify what success actually means, and what trade-offs may exist.

2. What Happens to Muscle During Weight Loss?

    - How much of the expected weight loss may come from muscle? (30-40% for all forms of weight loss)

- How will we monitor body composition, not just the number on the scale?

- What is my baseline muscle mass, and does that matter?

3. What Happens If I Stop the Medication?

- What do studies show about weight regain after discontinuation? (rapid and common)

- How quickly does regain typically occur? (regain ⅔ of the weight lost within a year)

- Does metabolism remain lower after weight loss? (Yes)

- Will we have a plan if I decide to stop? (???)

Understanding the likely trajectory reduces surprise and frustration later.

4. Is Long-Term Therapy Expected?

- Will I be taking this forever?

- What do we know (and not know) about multi-year or multi-decade use?

- What are the trade-offs between staying on the drug indefinitely vs. for a defined period of time?

5. Am I at Higher Risk for Muscle or Bone Loss?

- Am I older? Post-menopausal?

- Do I already have low muscle mass?

- Do I have osteopenia or osteoporosis?

- Have I dieted repeatedly in the past?

Some people are more vulnerable to structural shifts than others. Are you one of them?

6. What Will We Measure Beyond Weight?

- Will we track strength?
- Body composition?
- Bone health?
- Physical function?
- How often are our data points?

The Central Conversation

Starting a GLP-1 medication is not simply a decision to "lose weight" It is a decision to apply sustained pressure to a system that adapts. It may be appropriate and even life-changing, but it should be entered with open eyes.

The more clearly you understand how your body responds to change, the more intelligently you and your physician can decide together.

Bottom Line:

Your body does not "reset" after weight loss. It is physiologically reshaped by the weight loss itself.

When you lose weight, your metabolism often slows more than expected. Regain is therefore biologically predictable, not a moral failure.

GLP-1 medications can suppress appetite and support weight loss, and they also reconfigure metabolism and immunity in ways we do not fully understand.

During weight loss, whether through dieting, surgery or medication, muscle, bone, and metabolic rate may shift in ways that do not fully reverse.

Responsible use of these medications requires awareness of more than the number on the scale. It requires understanding how the whole system adapts.

****

Chapter 8

The words *health* and *whole* stem from the Proto-Indo-European root, *kailo-*, which meant "whole, uninjured, or of good omen," implying an inherent state of integrity. The root *kailo-* begat *holy*, suggesting that sacredness was borne of "wholeness".

Enough hails from a different lineage. It was sprung from the prefix *ġe-* and the root *nōg*, with *ġe-* traditionally indicating completeness, and *nōg* indicating sufficiency. But *Enough* is a restless child, ambitious and striving, always reaching. It hauls itself off its ass and climbs, just a little further, just *a bit more,* not quite ever *there* yet.

But *enough* can also be *no more*, a hard stop. *Enough* is a stopping rule that protects from intrusion and excess. It holds and stands its ground. This obstinacy is the muscle that prevents depletion. Disillusionment and burnout are the result of yielding to convenience and guilt. The drain of one-way relationships, the tyranny of escalating demands, the vine creep of work into uneasy weekends. We give in to wheedling, nagging, other people's expectations. Fatigue and anxiety erode our determination to say no; our resolve to stand our ground falls. Giving in is inevitable when we have forfeited our boundaries.

Normal internal rotation of the hip ranges from 30-45 degrees and mine was zero in the right hip. It didn't bother me for years but the more I danced the more my body tried to compensate. My pelvis tilted with the right side riding high and as my glutes took on the strain of overloading through hours of dancing and being on my feet, my hip flexors began to spasm from the strain of trying to compensate.

It wasn't until I couldn't dance anymore that I went to PT. I had to strengthen my glutes, I was told, and I approached that task like I was training for the Olympics. If I was assigned 2 sets of an exercise, I did 4. If my load was set at 10 lbs, why not 20? I can only see now that I was trying to deal with an overuse injury with...more overuse.

When Daniela met with me, she did a first rate assessment of my musculoskeletal alignment, but her approach surprised me. In one of our sessions she had me lie on my tummy with my right leg bent at the knee and up. With one hand on my lower back to stabilize me she held onto my leg and rocked it slowly back and forth in a windshield wiper motion. My only task was to focus on my breathing. For over thirty minutes she moved my leg in that slow arc, a gentle, rocking, motion that I relaxed into. At the end of the session, she was able to passively get my hip to 45 degrees of internal rotation.

It didn't last, of course. The minute I got on my feet, the tightness and limp returned. *It's not about doing more*, Daniela said, *it's about doing enough, and then letting your body process that before your next session*. This rattled me. While I was familiar with pushing myself, actively resisting doing anything was uncomfortable. Part of me knew she was right but it was hard to fully admit that I had been sabotaging my own recovery. Over the next weeks the full significance of her words seeped in. I needed to learn how to allow parts of my body to downshift and rest. It also spilled over into my thinking on how medicine is practised.

In over two decades as an obesity specialist, I have rarely encountered indifference. More often, I meet people who carry way more than their share. Parents balancing care for children and aging relatives. AM, an ICU nurse who later worked in oncology while supporting her family and caring for her brother. S, a patent lawyer who remained in a job environment he hated to provide stability for his family. D, a CNA working extended shifts to support her children. At work, accumulation is rewarded and expansion is progress as limits are negotiated or reframed. Over time, internal signals like hunger, satiety, fatigue, restoration—nudges from our body—become less decisive than external demands.

How could they do that to themselves? I was often asked about the patients I treated. As if they chose deliberate humiliation and shame, as if they plotted their ill health. These are not people lacking discipline. They are often the most reliable—those who step in, who absorb overflow, and keep systems running. Their days revolve around meeting the needs of others. What remains for themselves is often remnants of self-care in the form of convenience meals, irregular rest, and fragmented recovery. Our modern environment amplifies this pattern. Food is engineered for continued intake. Work is portable and unbounded, and stimulation constant. The conditions that once enforced limits such as seasonality and physical constraint are now negotiable.

Biology, however, has not changed at the same pace. Appetite, reward, and energy balance evolved in environments where boundaries were embedded in daily life. Meals, effort, and rest followed nature's rhythm. In April 2003, 92% of the human genome had been sequenced. By 2022, a complete human genome sequence was available. Over that same period, the prevalence of chronic disease in the United States rose from approximately 36–50% to over 75%. The number of Americans with two or more chronic conditions increased from 60 million to over 130 million.

We have focused on genetic causes of disease and deficiencies, while continuing to ignore the larger epigenetic causes. The tendency has been to alter our bodies to match the environment, and not the environment to match us. No-one asks what happens when biological systems shaped by constraint are placed in environments defined by excess. Much of what we call chronic disease may be the physiologic expression of sustained overflow—of systems operating without clear stopping points. Not a failure of will, but a mismatch between design and condition.

We live as if limits do not apply to us; we have made stopping optional. But what Daniela taught me is that rest is the body's reset, a natural phase of healing and repair. And as I continue my own journey to healing, I've learned the wisdom of restraint.

In recent years, a new term has quietly entered medical conversations around GLP-1 drugs: "micro-dosing." This is not in official prescribing guidelines nor is it a regulatory term but something some clinicians and patients have begun doing in practice.

Micro-dosing generally means taking a GLP-1 medication at a dose lower than the doses studied in major diabetes or obesity trials, and staying there (i.e. no dose escalation). For example, instead of escalating to full obesity doses, someone might remain at a very low weekly dose of semaglutide or tirzepatide. The idea is simple. Use just enough medication to soften hunger, but not enough to strongly suppress it.

How It Happened

When GLP-1 drugs were studied, researchers noticed something predictable: Higher doses produced greater weight loss and more nausea and side effects. Lower doses produced smaller weight loss but were easier to tolerate.

That is a classic dose–response curve. Some clinicians began asking *if a small dose produces some appetite control and fewer side effects, why push higher?* At the same time, another observation was becoming clear. When people stop GLP-1 therapy completely, weight often returns. So a second idea emerged. *What if we don't stop entirely but reduce to a small maintenance dose?*

Thus, micro-dosing became a middle ground that straddles full pharmacologic suppression of physiology and no drug therapy.

What Do We Actually Know?

From formal clinical trials, we know that lower doses of GLP-1 drugs produce modest weight loss while higher doses produce larger weight loss. Side effects increase with dose.

What we do *not* have are long-term trials designed to test chronic low-dose maintenance, muscle preservation and bone effects at low doses. Micro-dosing has not been formally studied as its own therapeutic category and remains an extrapolation from dose-response data.

The Word "Micro" Can Be Misleading

It sounds reassuring, but "micro" is relative to high pharmaceutical doses and not relative to your natural biology. Your body produces GLP-1 in brief pulses after meals with the natural hormone rising and falling within minutes.

Long-acting GLP-1 medications, even at low doses, are still supraphysiologic and remain in the bloodstream continuously for days. So while a lower dose may be a smaller pharmacologic signal, it still differs from physiologic pulsatility.

What People Report

In clinical forums and patient communities, common descriptions are: *It takes the edge off hunger*, *I just don't think about food as much*, and *I can stop before I'm stuffed*. Some people find they are able to maintain their weight without nausea or other side effects.

These reports are consistent with what we know about lower doses. Smaller signal → smaller appetite suppression → fewer side effects. What is not being measured in these anecdotes are body composition (fat vs. muscle), resting metabolic rate, long-term adaptation of hunger pathways, bone density and inflammatory signaling. That's hardly surprising as most conversations center on hunger and scale weight, not systemic physiology. (That's not so different from the official drug trials, by the way, or even standard clinical care.)

When modest appetite control is the goal

In clinical practice, the weight loss associated with micro-dosing GLP-1 medications is usually modest. Many physicians report outcomes such as five to ten pounds of weight loss, sometimes even less.

At this level of dosing, the effect is subtle rather than dramatic. Appetite may be softened, but it is rarely eliminated. This pattern is consistent with what researchers see in dose–response studies, i.e. smaller doses produce smaller behavioral and metabolic effects.

Given that the effect is modest, if the goal is simply to reduce appetite slightly, why not use one of the older appetite suppressants?

Phentermine: an old drug with a long history

One of the oldest medications used for appetite suppression is phentermine, a sympathomimetic drug that was approved by the FDA in 1959 for short-term weight management. Phentermine works primarily by increasing norepinephrine/noradrenaline signaling in the hypothalamus, which suppresses appetite and reduces food intake.

Despite its age, the drug still produces measurable weight loss. A systematic review of older trials reported a mean total weight loss of about 6.3 kg (~14 lbs), with approximately 3.6 kg (~8 lbs) more weight loss than placebo in studies lasting between 2 and 24 weeks. Other reviews summarize typical results more conservatively as roughly 3–8% body-weight reduction, depending on dose, duration, and study population.

These numbers place phentermine in the same general territory as what many patients experience with very low doses of GLP-1 medications: modest appetite suppression and modest weight reduction. Yet the two drugs are often perceived very differently. Understanding why requires looking at both physiology, psychology, and perhaps, marketing.

The reputation of phentermine versus the data

Phentermine carries a long-standing reputation as a stimulant drug that can raise blood pressure and heart rate. Because it is sympathomimetic (stimulates the sympathetic nervous system), this concern is theoretically reasonable. But the average cardiovascular signal seen in obesity studies has often been smaller than many clinicians expect.

In one observational study examining long-term phentermine therapy, investigators found that treatment was not associated with increases in systolic blood pressure, diastolic blood pressure, or heart rate, and that many patients actually experienced improvements in blood-pressure categories, probably due to weight loss. While this does not mean phentermine (or any drug) is risk-free, its real-world negative cardiovascular effects are often less dramatic than its reputation suggests.

Current labeling for phentermine use in pregnancy advises against using phentermine during pregnancy because weight loss itself is not considered beneficial during pregnancy, not because a clear teratogenic signal has been demonstrated. In a prospective cohort study of women exposed to phentermine/fenfluramine during the first trimester, there was no increased rate of major structural birth defects, although they did find a higher rate of gestational diabetes in the exposed group. Other summaries of available data note that current human evidence has not demonstrated a clear increase in birth-defect risk, while also emphasizing that the dataset is limited.

Why are we less concerned about ADHD stimulants?

At this point, a curious asymmetry becomes visible.

FDA labeling for ADHD medications such as Adderall XR and Concerta explicitly states that stimulant medications can increase blood pressure by about 2–4 mmHg and heart rate by roughly 3–6 beats per minute on average. (As an example, if your baseline blood pressure and heart rate are 130/60 and 75, they can potentially be increased to 134/60 and 81). These effects are well known and routinely monitored.

Yet these medications are widely prescribed, and the modest hemodynamic changes they produce are generally accepted as part of their risk–benefit profile. Phentermine, by contrast, is often treated with greater suspicion, even though the average cardiovascular signal in obesity studies is not clearly larger.

Part of the difference is pharmacologic, but part of it is cultural. ADHD medications are framed as treatments for a recognized neurobehavioral disorder. Phentermine still carries the historical label of a "diet pill." The stigma surrounding obesity treatment has shaped how the drug is perceived.

Drug Scheduling: Phentermine vs Adderall

One of the reasons phentermine still carries stigma is that it belongs to a category of drugs known as controlled substances. These medications are regulated under the U.S. Controlled Substances Act because they have the potential for misuse or dependence. Controlled drugs are placed into *schedules*, which reflect the government's judgment about their medical usefulness and abuse potential. The categories run from Schedule I to Schedule V.

Schedule	Meaning
Schedule I	No accepted medical use; high abuse potential
Schedule II	Accepted medical use; high abuse potential
Schedule III–V	Accepted medical use; progressively lower abuse potential

The two drugs discussed here fall into different schedules:

- **Phentermine** → Schedule **IV**

- **Adderall (mixed amphetamine salts)** → Schedule **II**

Phentermine: Schedule IV

Phentermine is classified as a Schedule IV controlled substance.

This category includes medications with **lower abuse potential** than drugs in Schedules II or III. Despite being relatively low on the controlled-substance hierarchy, phentermine's reputation has remained colored by its history as a "diet pill."

Adderall: Schedule II

Adderall, which contains mixed amphetamine salts, is classified as a Schedule II controlled substance. This category includes medications with **high abuse potential**, though they still have accepted medical uses.

Other Schedule II drugs include morphine, oxycodone, fentanyl, and methylphenidate (Ritalin, Concerta). So Adderall is on the same schedule as opiates.

The Curious Contrast

Here is where the comparison becomes interesting. Even though Adderall is placed in a stricter schedule than phentermine, the two drugs are perceived very differently. Adderall and related ADHD medications are widely accepted as legitimate treatments for a recognized neurobehavioral disorder. Millions of prescriptions are written every year.

Phentermine, by contrast, is often approached with more hesitation, even though its schedule indicates lower abuse potential, and the average cardiovascular signal seen in obesity studies is modest. This difference illustrates how medical narratives shape prescribing behavior.

Phentermine vs. Adderall

Feature	Phentermine	Adderall (mixed amphetamine salts)
Controlled-substance schedule	Schedule IV	Schedule II
Abuse potential (DEA classification)	• lower abuse potential relative to Schedule II/III	• high abuse potential
Accepted medical use	• short-term obesity treatment	• ADHD • narcolepsy
Refills allowed?	• yes • ≤5 refills within 6 months (federal rule)	• no refills allowed
Typical prescription supply	• often ≤30 days • some clinicians prescribe longer intervals depending on state law	• typically ≤30 days
Prescription format	• written • electronic • sometimes telephone (state dependent)	• written or electronic only • stricter monitoring
Clinical monitoring expectations	• BP & HR monitoring recommended	• BP & HR monitoring recommended
Common clinical perception	• often labeled "diet pill" • sometimes viewed with caution	• widely accepted ADHD therapy
Approx. annual U.S. prescriptions	• ~7–9 million	• ~30–40 million

Prescription Volume in the United States

Prescription data also illustrate how common ADHD stimulant use has become. Here are the approximate annual U.S. prescription volumes in recent years.

Drug	Estimated annual prescriptions
Adderall / amphetamine stimulants	~30–40 million prescriptions
Phentermine	~7–9 million prescriptions*

*A 2025 JAMA Network Open analysis reported phentermine at about **0.74 million monthly prescriptions by February 2024**, which annualizes to roughly 8–9 million if sustained, but annual totals vary by source and year.

Despite being an older drug with modest cost and measurable effectiveness, phentermine is prescribed far less often than ADHD stimulants. There is cultural stigma around weight-loss drugs ("diet pills") and theoretical concern about stimulants in obesity treatment. The emergence of newer drugs such as GLP-1 receptor agonists have also pushed it into the shadows.

A Perspective Worth Considering

Phentermine and Adderall are not equivalent drugs but the contrast does highlight an important point. Medical comfort with a medication often reflects history, culture, and expectations, not just pharmacology and outcomes. A stimulant used for ADHD may be accepted despite measurable effects on blood pressure and heart rate. Meanwhile, a sympathomimetic used for weight management may remain controversial even when its average physiological effects are modest. Recognizing these differences in perception helps clarify how treatment decisions are shaped, not only by science, but also by narrative.

So let's go back to my question of why there is a preference for micro-dosing GLP-1 drugs instead of phentermine. With GLP-1 microdosing, the expected outcome is often a small reduction in appetite and several pounds of weight loss rather than dramatic metabolic change. When the magnitude of benefit is this limited, the comparison landscape widens. Cost, tolerability, accessibility, and real-world persistence begin to matter as much as mechanism.

Cost: the most practical difference

Generic phentermine is inexpensive. Through common discount programs, a month's supply can cost roughly $12–$16.

GLP-1 medications exist in an entirely different pricing universe. The official U.S. list price for Wegovy (semaglutide 2.4 mg) is $1,349.02 per package, although manufacturer programs and insurance coverage can sometimes reduce the monthly out-of-pocket cost to roughly $149–$349 for some patients.

Over-the-counter orlistat (Alli), another weight loss medication, typically costs around $50–$60 per month.

When the weight-loss effect of micro-dosing is modest, this price difference becomes hard to ignore.

A Question Worth Asking

If micro-dosed GLP-1 therapy produces modest appetite suppression and modest weight reduction, why not use older medications such as phentermine, which are inexpensive and well studied?

Several factors may contribute to the preference for GLP-1–based approaches. First, GLP-1 receptor agonists are framed as *metabolic hormone therapies*, whereas phentermine is historically associated with stimulant appetite suppression and the era of "diet pills." This difference in narrative shapes clinician comfort and patient expectations.

Second, GLP-1 drugs have demonstrated broader metabolic benefits, including improvements in glycemic control and cardiovascular outcomes in patients with diabetes. Third, side-effect profiles differ. Phentermine's possible side effects are insomnia, anxiety, or palpitations in susceptible individuals, while GLP-1 therapies more commonly produce GI symptoms such as nausea.

Finally, the current momentum of obesity pharmacotherapy strongly favors incretin-based therapies, which are perceived as part of a newer generation of metabolic treatments. Even so, the comparison highlights an important point: medical decisions are shaped not only by pharmacology and outcomes but also by history, culture, and expectations.

Phentermine remains an inexpensive sympathomimetic medication capable of producing modest but measurable weight loss, typically in the range of 3–8% of body weight. GLP-1 receptor agonists produce substantially greater weight loss at full therapeutic doses but often yield smaller reductions in real-world settings, particularly when lower doses are used.

Micro-dosing strategies represent an attempt to balance efficacy, tolerability, and affordability, but the long-term metabolic consequences of sustained low-level receptor stimulation remain uncertain. Understanding how these therapies compare, both mechanistically and in terms of real-world outcomes, helps clarify the broader landscape of obesity pharmacotherapy.

GLP-1: Trials versus the Real World

The success of GLP-1 medications in clinical trials has been striking. In the STEP-1 trial, semaglutide 2.4 mg (full-dose) produced average weight loss of about 14.9% at 68 weeks, with 4.5% of participants discontinuing because of gastrointestinal side effects.

In the SURMOUNT-1 trial, tirzepatide produced mean weight loss ranging from 15.0% to 20.9% at 72 weeks, depending on the dose used. Discontinuation due to adverse events ranged from 4.3% to 7.1%.

Under carefully controlled trial conditions, these drugs clearly work. But real-world use often looks different. In a large Cleveland Clinic study involving 7,881 patients, the average one-year weight reduction was 8.7% overall. Outcomes varied significantly depending on whether patients stayed on treatment:

- 3.6% weight loss with early discontinuation
- 6.8% weight loss with later discontinuation
- 11.9% weight loss among those who remained on therapy

Importantly, **80.8% of patients were using lower doses**, not the full trial dose.

In other words, once the complexities of everyday life enter the picture—cost, side effects, insurance issues, and patient preferences—real-world results often become more modest than the headline numbers from clinical trials.

Comparison of Drug Costs

Drug	Approximate U.S. cost	Common limiting factors	Real-world use
Phentermine	About $12 to $16 per month with discount pricing	Insomnia, dry mouth, stimulant reputation, disappointment with modest loss	Long-term use common in practice despite short-term FDA approval
Semaglutide 2.4 mg (Wegovy)	List price about $1,349 per month; some self-pay programs about $149 to $349 per month	Nausea, vomiting, GI intolerance, cost, insurance barriers	Large cohort: 8.7% average weight loss at 1 year; 80.8% maintained on lower doses
Tirzepatide (Zepbound class)	Premium branded pricing	GI side effects, cost, adherence	Real-world results reduced by discontinuation and dose reduction
Orlistat (Alli)	About $50 to $60 per month OTC	Oily stool, fecal urgency, spotting, steatorrhea	Frequent discontinuation despite OTC availability

A Conceptual Insight: Energy Deficit Rather Than Mechanism

These comparisons highlight an important principle of metabolic physiology. Weight loss ultimately reflects sustained energy deficit, regardless of the pharmacologic pathway used to achieve it. Different medications influence appetite and metabolism through distinct mechanisms. Phentermine increases catecholamine signaling within hypothalamic appetite circuits, while GLP-1 receptor agonists activate incretin pathways that regulate satiety and insulin secretion.

Yet if two treatments produce similar net reductions in caloric intake, their weight-loss trajectories may converge. The plateau occurs when energy expenditure and energy intake reach a new equilibrium. From this perspective, the magnitude of the pharmacologic signal may matter as much as the mechanism itself. A powerful intervention can sustain weight loss over a longer trajectory before plateau, whereas a smaller intervention may stabilize earlier.

This framework helps explain why the modest appetite suppression produced by micro-dosed GLP-1 therapy may lead to weight loss in the same general range historically observed with stimulant appetite suppressants.

What Happens in Real Patients

Clinical trials tell us what medications can do under controlled conditions. Real-world practice often tells a different story.

Over the years, I prescribed phentermine to appropriate patients with good weight loss results. Even then, what I observed was not dramatic failures or dangerous side effects, but something more mundane: people often stopped the medication for reasons that had little to do with pharmacology. In my experience, **almost all my patients stopped before vacations or holidays** despite my counseling. They would tell me quite openly that they wanted to enjoy the food while traveling or celebrating with family. The medication was not the problem. The timing simply conflicted with how they wanted to live.

Others stopped because they felt the drug "wasn't doing much." When we looked more closely, the medication had produced measurable effects. Appetite was dampened and they had lost 6-10 pounds, with beneficial improvements in blood sugar and heart health. The issue was not that the drug had no effect but that the effect did not match what they imagined. Expectations had outrun biology.

In medical practice, phentermine is not prescribed for aesthetic weight loss. The medication is generally used for individuals with obesity or obesity-related health risks. Yet culturally, the category of "diet pills" became associated with cosmetic weight loss in earlier decades, when over-the-counter products such as Dexatrim were widely marketed. People who used those products discovered something very quickly: once they stopped taking the pills, their weight returned.

This experience should not surprise us. Appetite suppressants do not change the basic physiology of weight regulation; they temporarily modify it. When the drug is removed, the biological pressures that favor weight regain reassert themselves. There is little reason to believe this principle will be fundamentally different with GLP-1 receptor agonists. These medications influence powerful metabolic and appetite pathways, but they do not erase the underlying biology of weight regulation. As with earlier appetite suppressants, stopping treatment often leads to some degree of weight regain.

My patients and I were always *real* with each other. I appreciated and respected their honesty and we all learned together that obesity is a formidable disease because of its physiologic, social and emotional complexity. A drug is just one tool, as are meal replacements and surgery. What we are fighting is how to live in a world where technology and convenience have outstripped our biological capacity to adapt. Our bodies are not enough for the rapidly-arriving future worlds that outrun our development.

Recognizing this helps place the newer drugs into perspective. The pharmacology may be more sophisticated, but the broader behavioral and physiological dynamics are yet to be addressed.

Bottom Line

Micro-dosing is not reckless or irrational but it has not been formally validated. It does represent a common pattern in medicine in that practice evolves before research catches up. For some individuals, low doses may provide meaningful appetite control with fewer side effects.

What remains uncertain is the long-term metabolic cost — or neutrality — of maintaining even a small external signal in systems that evolved around rhythmic internal ones.

****

Chapter 9

Heartbreak warps the heart.

A dating recession has developed over the last two decades and over 40% of adults in the country are now unpartnered. Financial strain and social stress are part of the picture, but those of us who have loved and lost are more cautious. We learn the defence of needing less. In the body, scar tissue changes the heart's architecture and, in doing so, weakens its pumping. In love, heartbreak and grief reshape our lives even as we heal.

Elsewhere, Hammerhead worms are mostly reproducing through fission. They divide themselves into fragments, each piece regenerating into a complete organism. Trying to kill a Hammerhead worm by cutting it only creates more of them. In some regions, entire populations are clones—genetic copies, proliferating without the need for another. No courtship or rejection, no loss. It is a life that has eliminated the problem of needing the other, snug in its self-sufficiency.

We are not so different. Human reproduction is declining across developed countries. In its place, artificial systems proliferate in the form of AI replicas, digital avatars, and endless self-generated content. We can now produce without friction and generate without waiting, in a virtual mode increasingly composed of ourselves. Welcome to a paradoxical world of excess and lack where biological systems rooted in the constraints of the physical world are overridden for diminishing returns.

I wonder if the worms are lonely. Talking to your other half may not be as interesting when it literally is *your other half*. What do worms do when they only have themselves? Do they get bored and mindlessly hunt snails or earthworms just for fun? Would snacking on their prey relieve the isolation? In their desperation do they fragment into pieces of themselves just to have a friend?

Ah, and the heart.

Fibroblasts lay down collagen to seal a wound. It is fast, efficient, and lifesaving. Scar tissue is for surviving because even dysfunction is a sign of life. Eating, too, can become a way of sealing over absence, stabilizing a system that no longer trusts what comes from the outside. In my clinic, I sit across from patients who are not alone, and yet profoundly lonely. They speak of loss and disconnection, of a gradual retreat from intimacy. In the absence of what once nourished them, food becomes a kind of repair.

Hammerhead worms are invading the earth. They hitchhike through soil and root systems in nurseries and gardens, multiplying as they fragment, each generation further removed from its origin. We're not so different from worms. We know how to go on producing within the narrow straits of the self.

By this point in the book, it should be clear that GLP-1 medications are not simply "weight-loss drugs." They enter a complex immune-metabolic system, alter appetite and signaling, change body weight and body composition, and may affect people differently depending on physiology, context, comorbidities, nutrition, strength, and time horizon. For that reason, the practical question is not merely whether to start, continue, or stop a GLP-1 medication. but how to make these decisions thoughtfully.

This chapter offers a framework for that process. It is not a substitute for individualized medical care, and it is not a universal protocol. Instead, it is a way to organize the questions that should be asked before starting treatment, while continuing treatment, and when considering dose reduction or stopping. The goal is not simply to lose weight. The goal is to protect health, preserve function, reduce avoidable risk, and make the medication serve the person rather than letting the number on the scale become the only measure of success.

Before You Start the Medication

Starting a GLP-1 medication is not just about losing weight. It is a decision to temporarily override your appetite biology. Before beginning, you should understand why you are taking it (blood sugar? heart risk? weight-related complications?), what you are hoping to change, and what trade-offs may come with long-term use.

Ask your physician:

- What is my actual medical indication?
- What are my muscle and bone risks?
- Do I need a baseline body composition scan (DXA)?
- What is our long-term plan — stay on, reduce later, or reassess?

What to Establish While You're On It (Even Better, Before You Begin)

GLP-1 medications suppress appetite. They don't build muscle, strengthen bone or automatically improve fitness. While your hunger is lower, you must actively protect your muscle mass, bone and your nutrition.

Protein

Most adults on therapy should aim for roughly **25–30 grams of whole-food protein per meal**, unless their physician advises otherwise. In practice, this is easier than calculating grams per kilogram of body weight or lean mass, and it helps create clear protein pulses across the day. This usually means having a clear source of (preferably animal-based, such as eggs, dairy, meat) protein at every meal, and not skipping meals simply because you are not hungry. Aim for at least 3 meals a day.

Resistance Training

Muscle is preserved by load, not by intention. At minimum you should have 2-3 sessions of resistance training per week. The exercises should challenge major muscle groups and should increase in exertion level over time.

Alcohol

Alcohol is a Group 1 carcinogen, which means there is no safe lower limit. In a catabolic state with reduced intake, alcohol displaces protein. Because of its toxicity your body metabolizes the alcohol first before any other macronutrient. This allows you to neutralize its damaging effects by burning alcohol for fuel before anything else. Alcohol worsens muscle health by impairing recovery after workouts.

The medical recommendation should be clear: No alcohol. But just like smoking, the choice is yours.

Understanding Weight Loss vs Body Composition

Not all weight loss is fat. During GLP-1 therapy, some portion of weight lost is muscle. In clinical trials, approximately 25% to 40% of total weight lost was lean mass. If you lose 40 pounds, 10–16 pounds may be muscle. If you regain 40 lbs, most of it will likely be fat. So besides strength, balance and metabolic stability, muscle is important in long-term weight maintenance.

Since the scale does not tell the whole story, ask your physician about:

- Body composition tracking (DXA)
- Strength measurements
- Functional testing

What Happens If You Stop

Clinical studies show that when people stop these medications, significant weight regain is common, with ⅔ of people regaining 75% of the total weight lost within the year. So if you lose 40 pounds and stop the drug, one year later your total weight loss would be ~10 lbs, even with maintenance of healthy lifestyle behaviors. Two years out from stopping the medication, many will likely be at their initial (pre-weight loss) baseline weight.

This reflects biological counter-regulation. This is why you need to have clear discussions about medication goals and your exit strategy even before you begin using these drugs. While the trial data and advertising scripts may be impressive, make sure you align your expectations to real world data so as not to be blindsided during your journey. Keep in mind that if you lost 60 pounds, long-term maintenance off medication may realistically be closer to 15 pounds (25% of total weight lost), according to a large meta-analysis.

Long-Term Use is a Decision to be Made with Your Doctor

Long-term use is not "set it and forget it." Your doctor should periodically reassess:

- Do benefits still outweigh potential long-term trade-offs?
- Are you preserving muscle?
- Are you metabolically stable?

The fact that a medication works does not mean it should be continued indefinitely without reassessment.

If You and Your Doctor Decide to Lower the Dose

Dose reduction should be gradual and you should know that as the medication decreases, hunger may increase. Instead of abruptly stopping, consider replacing medication with more meal structure as you wean down on your doses.

This can be done by increasing to 3-5 meals a day, adding additional protein-based meals as needed, spacing meals roughly 3 hours apart. Ensure each meal contains meaningful whole animal protein, and increase fiber and whole-food volume for satiety.

You are replacing pharmacologic appetite control with behavioral architecture in order to help reduce rebound weight gain. By now you should have a regular routine of resistance training which should be continued. Track your weight changes, hunger patterns and muscle strength. If weight increases rapidly and persistently, you might need your dose adjusted by your doctor. If you need help with implementing structure, I have designed a Guide and Workbook plus live Q&A sessions to take you through the practical steps involved.

Muscle Matters More Than You Think

Over time, especially with aging, it becomes harder to rebuild muscle. Without adequate stimulus body composition may worsen even if weight looks "acceptable." Whether you stay on the medication or not, muscle preservation is non-negotiable.

***If you would like a deeper guide to the science of preserving muscle, go to Wellth-e.com[1] and check out **Issue 3: New Insights to Muscle Health**: https://wellth-e.com/2026/01/11/issue-3-overview/

Bottom Line

These medications can improve blood sugar and reduce weight but they do not permanently reset appetite biology. Being on them does not replace exercise or eliminate the need for nutritional discipline

****

1. http://wellth-e.com

Chapter 10

I used to be part of a rabbit rescue. Rabbits are domestic animals and should never be released in the wild. Despite this, we took in dozens and dozens of these abandoned pets every year, particularly after Easter. People had a hard time understanding that domestically bred rabbits were not the same as wild ones and would never survive on their own.

One of my favourite breeds was the Floppy Eared Rabbit and I've rescued several of them. Their long hanging ears and round face give them an endearing look that makes them so appealing. But as with human aesthetics, these sought-after features come with a price. I had to learn very quickly that lop-eared rabbits are some of the most difficult pets because of their health risks.

Rabbits use their erect ears to regulate their body temperatures, so drooping ears impair airflow and heat dissipation, making them prone to hyperthermia. Their ears are also difficult to groom, resulting in mites and wax that not only compromise their hearing but make them prone to balance issues and head tilt disease. Any rabbit owner who has ever had to care for a bunny with head tilt will know the stress and grief of watching your beloved pet struggle to move, eat and drink.

Anhui was a quiet bunny, reserved compared to my other rescues. And when she developed head tilt disease, I stayed up with her all night to comfort her. The hardest thing was having to leave her to go to work, knowing she would spend the day with one cheek on the ground, her head twisted from a disease that was also called wry neck. She lay there, eyes rolling from vertigo, and when she moved she would fall and roll over, legs thrashing in the air to regain balance. I padded her enclosure, the floor, all hard surfaces, and tried to place a cushion beneath her cheek as she lay there grinding her teeth.

Besides their distinctive ears, their round faces are due to selective breeding for brachycephaly, a condition that flattens their faces for that 'cute' look. This leads to significant painful dental disease that may shorten their lifespans. I've had bunnies with dental spurs, abscesses and malocclusion where the upper and lower teeth do not line up, resulting in the inability to grind the tooth surfaces properly. Their 'cuteness' made them popular in pet stores but when their health deteriorated they were abandoned, often let loose 'to be free', but more certainly, to their death.

This is not unique to rabbits. *Homo sapiens* has effectively been domesticating itself for millenia. From the technology of fire we learned to cook, and our jaws and digestive tracts shrank. Dairy farming selected for lactose-digesting enzymes in Northern Europe and parts of Africa. Antibiotics have reshaped our immune systems. And our outsourcing of memory, navigation and thinking to digital devices is restructuring the brain such that we might eventually be impaired rather than inconvenienced without a digital interface.

As we continue to manipulate our environments and bodies, gene-culture coevolution will become more and more prominent in the development of our species. In doing so we may echo *Frankenstein*'s Creature: "If I cannot satisfy the one, I will indulge the other."

And perhaps we will also hear the unease of its maker, Victor Frankenstein: "How dangerous is the acquirement of knowledge, and how much happier that man is who believes his native town to be the world, than **he who aspires to become greater than his nature will allow**."

This chapter is intended primarily **for physicians** and other licensed health professionals. It will also be illuminating for readers who want a clearer view of how medical judgment is formed, and cautionary for those considering "self-managing" these medications after obtaining them through online or otherwise fragmented systems of care.

Access to a prescription is not the same as receiving thoughtful medical care, and these decisions involve far more than weight or dose escalation. The movement from evidence to treatment is never automatic, and the movement from weight loss to health is not straightforward. Real judgment asks more of us. It asks us to consider body composition, nutritional sufficiency, comorbidity, symptoms, inflammatory state, tolerance, and time horizon. It asks us to think not only about whether something works, but what kind of change it produces, for whom, and at what cost.

Between evidence and action lies judgment. This chapter is about that difficult middle space, where medicine cannot be reduced to a protocol, a platform, or a number on a scale.

Why this chapter exists

Most physicians first "meet" a new drug in one of three ways: a glossy supplement from a journal, a conference talk, or a rep's slide deck with a handful of hazard ratios and p-values. By the time the drug reaches us, the evidence has already been compressed into a narrative: this class reduces risk by X%, is safe, and should be used in patients like yours. I'd like to use this chapter to pull that process apart.

Drug trials are not neutral mirrors of reality. They are instruments built for specific purposes: to satisfy regulators, convince payers, and generate a coherent marketing story. They answer narrowly defined questions in narrowly defined populations over relatively short periods of time. That is not a flaw but the nature of the tool.

The problem arises when **we forget what the tool was built to do** and use it as if it had answered questions it never even asked. A cardiovascular outcome trial can tell you something about MACE over 3–5 years in high-risk patients but it cannot tell you what 15 years of pharmacologic weight suppression does to muscle, bone, neurocognition, infection tolerance, or survivorship after cancer. It can show you a statistically significant relative risk reduction but it cannot, by itself, tell you whether that absolute benefit meets *this* patient's threshold for "worth it," or what is being traded away to obtain it.

With GLP-1 receptor agonists, these gaps become particularly stark. We now have proof of meaningful weight loss and cardiovascular benefit in select populations, with emerging signals about lean mass loss, potential effects on bone, and complex immune-metabolic interactions. There is still very little long-term, body-composition and frailty-aware outcome data in the time frames that actually matter for an aging population already living with anabolic resistance.

The central message of this chapter is simple: **Evidence is necessary but not sufficient.** *Judgment* is what we do with the evidence, the biology, the patient in front of us, and the uncertainties the trials leave behind. Our professional responsibility is not to be passive recipients of "data" but active interpreters. Our role is to see what was measured and what was omitted; to translate relative risk into absolute terms; to ask what happens to muscle, bone, brain, and immune resilience when we extend a short-term trial paradigm into decades of real life.

In an era where AI systems can summarize guidelines and parse PDFs faster than any of us, this interpretive, skeptical, integrative work is the part of medicine that cannot be automated away. This need for clinical judgement is what preserves the physician's value in the age of AI.

Scope and constraints

The goal is not to foster cynicism about an industry or nihilism about pharmacotherapy. Instead I want to provide practical mental tools: ways of reading a paper, sanity-checking a hazard ratio, interrogating an endpoint list, and integrating muscle, bone, function, and "hidden hunger" into decisions about long-term GLP-1 use.

Within this frame, the chapter will:

- Examine what drug trials are designed to do (and not do)

- Contrast relative and absolute risk, and how their presentation shapes both physician and patient choices

- Situate GLP-1–associated lean mass loss within the broader biology of anabolic resistance, frailty, and mortality

- Revisit "hunger" through the lenses of brain perfusion and nutrient-specific appetite

- Raise specific questions about stacking GLP-1 therapy on top of bariatric surgery

- Argue for a conception of the physician's role that goes beyond "following guidelines" to stewardship of long-term functional reserve

Everything that follows is an invitation for physicians to re-claim that role, to move from evidence to judgment in a way that is explicit, transparent, and worthy of the trust patients place in us.

What Drug Trials Are Made To Do, And What They Are Not

Modern large drug trials, including cardiovascular outcome trials (CVOTs), are regulatory instruments. After the 2008 FDA guidance requiring demonstration of cardiovascular safety for new glucose-lowering agents, sponsors were compelled to design large, event-driven trials powered to assess major adverse cardiovascular events (MACE). These typically include a composite of:

- Cardiovascular death

- Non-fatal myocardial infarction

- Non-fatal stroke

Sometimes this is expanded to include hospitalization for unstable angina or heart failure. Key design characteristics of GLP-1 CVOTs (e.g., LEADER, SUSTAIN-6, REWIND, etc.) include:

- High baseline cardiovascular risk populations

- Median follow-up ~2–5 years

- Event-driven stopping rules

- Time-to-event analysis using hazard ratios

These trials are explicitly powered to detect **relative risk differences** between groups for predefined composite endpoints. They are not designed to:

- Detect long-term effects beyond the study duration

- Fully characterize body composition trajectories (DXA often limited to substudies)

- Evaluate frailty progression, sarcopenia incidence, or bone density as primary outcomes

- Capture downstream stress tolerance (infection survival, chemotherapy tolerance, surgical resilience)

The statistical architecture reflects this purpose: large N, pre-specified endpoints, hierarchical testing procedures to protect type I error, and time-to-event Cox proportional hazards models. This is appropriate for regulatory approval. It is not equivalent to answering *what happens to this physiology over decades?*

Composite Endpoints: Power vs Interpretation

Composite endpoints are used to increase statistical power and reduce required sample size by aggregating multiple events. Advantages:

- Faster accrual of events

- Increased ability to detect statistical differences

- Regulatory efficiency

Limitations:

- Components may not be equally clinically meaningful

- A reduction in a softer endpoint (e.g., hospitalization) can dominate the composite

- Relative risk reduction may be driven primarily by one component while others remain unchanged

For example, in some CVOTs, separation curves are largely driven by reductions in non-fatal events, while cardiovascular mortality differences may be smaller or non-significant. The composite hazard ratio, however, is what is most often communicated.

Clinically, this means that a 13% relative reduction in MACE does not automatically translate into a 13% reduction in cardiovascular death, nor does it specify which component is driving the effect. The composite endpoint statistically compresses nuance.

Relative Risk as the Native Language of Trials

Most large outcome trials report:

- Hazard ratio (HR)

- Relative risk reduction (RRR)

- Confidence intervals

- p-values

Relative risk is mathematically stable across populations of differing baseline risk. This is precisely why it is favored in regulatory science. However, **absolute risk reduction (ARR) is a function of baseline risk.** If baseline 5-year event risk is:

- 20%, a 15% relative reduction produces a 3% absolute reduction.

- 10%, the same 15% relative reduction produces a 1.5% absolute reduction.

- 5%, it produces a 0.75% absolute reduction.

The trial may report a hazard ratio of 0.85 in all three cases. Clinically, these are very different realities.

Number Needed to Treat (NNT) depends entirely on ARR, not RRR. Yet relative risk reduction is visually and rhetorically more compelling. A "15% reduction" sounds large. A "1.5% absolute reduction over 5 years" feels smaller. Both are true, and which one the physician mentally prioritizes changes practice.

Duration, Discontinuation, and the Silence of the Long Horizon

Most GLP-1 CVOTs have median follow-up periods of 2–5 years. Weight-loss trials (e.g., STEP program) generally range from 68 weeks to 2 years, with some extension data. What we do not yet have:

- 10–20 year randomized data on chronic GLP-1 exposure
- Longitudinal frailty trajectories
- Sarcopenia incidence as a primary endpoint
- Cumulative bone mineral density outcomes over decades
- Data on what happens after repeated cycles of initiation and discontinuation

Absence of evidence is not evidence of harm, **and** not evidence of safety across long time horizons. When therapy is intended to be lifelong, the duration of evidence matters.

Trial Design Shapes Narrative

It is essential to acknowledge that trial design decisions shape interpretation. Examples include:

- Selecting high-risk populations (increases event rate → magnifies absolute benefit)

- Using run-in periods that exclude non-adherent or intolerant patients

- Defining rescue criteria in ways that influence comparator group outcomes

- Stopping trials at pre-specified interim analyses once significance thresholds are met

All of these are legitimate design strategies but they are not neutral. They create a specific evidentiary frame, i.e., one that maximizes clarity for a particular regulatory question. Clinical medicine operates outside that frame.

Takeaway

Drug trials are engineered tools. They are designed to detect statistically significant relative differences in predefined endpoints over limited time horizons in specific populations. They are not designed to:

- Fully characterize long-term physiologic trade-offs

- Capture body composition consequences over decades

- Resolve value judgments about acceptable benefit thresholds

- Substitute for individualized risk translation

Understanding what a trial was built to answer is the first step toward responsible interpretation.

Relative vs Absolute Risk: Why Relative Risk Dominates the Conversation

Most large outcome trials report results in the form of:

- Hazard ratio (HR)

- Relative risk reduction (RRR)

- Confidence intervals

- p-values

A hazard ratio of 0.85 is typically translated into *a 15% reduction in major adverse cardiovascular events.* This is technically correct but incomplete and potentially deceptive.

Relative risk reduction answers the question *by what proportion did events decrease relative to the control group?* It does **not** answer *how many fewer people actually experienced an event?* That second question is answered by **absolute risk reduction (ARR)**. And that is where clinical decisions live.

The Same Relative Risk, Different Realities

Consider a simplified example using numbers consistent with major CVOT ranges:

If 5-year event rate in placebo = 20%

If HR = 0.85

Then:

- Treatment group event rate ≈ 17%

- Absolute risk reduction = 3%

- NNT ≈ 33 over 5 years

Now let's reduce baseline risk:

If placebo event rate = 10%

Same HR = 0.85

Then:

- Treatment event rate ≈ 8.5%

- Absolute risk reduction = 1.5%

- NNT ≈ 67 over 5 years

Same hazard ratio, double the NNT. This is not statistical trickery, just mathematics. Yet hazard ratios are portable across populations; absolute risk is not. That is why trials emphasize RRR. **Clinical practice, however, is population-specific and patient-specific.**

Table 10.1–Same Relative Risk, Different Absolute Impact (10-Year Horizon)

Baseline 10-yr Risk	Relative Risk Reduction	Absolute Risk Reduction	NNT (10 yrs)
20%	25%	5%	20
10%	25%	2.5%	40
5%	25%	1.25%	80
2%	25%	0.5%	200

Relative risk is statistically stable while absolute risk is what is clinically meaningful. When we fail to translate hazard ratios into absolute terms, we inadvertently magnify perceived benefit.

Statins as the Template

The statin literature provides a well-characterized example of this dynamic. Major statin trials and subsequent meta-analyses demonstrate:

- ~20–30% relative reduction in major vascular events

- More modest absolute reductions depending on baseline risk

Let's take the ASCOT-LLA trial. It was designed to look at primary prevention in a high risk population of patients with hypertension but no prior heart disease using the drug, atorvastatin, at 10 mg a day. The primary end-point was non-fatal MI and also fatal heart disease. This was reported as a RRR of 36% and many health organizations have run away with this, demanding that all their healthcare providers prescribe statins across the board to patients to prevent atherosclerotic heart disease per lipid panel criteria, specifically total cholesterol and LDL-C levels. Some of you in primary care might even have been ding-ed by your healthcare system for not clicking that 'prescribe' button every time you come across a "high cholesterol" or "high-LDL-C" number.

What these systems failed to note was that even in this high-risk population, the ARR was 1.1%, requiring treatment of 91 such high risk patients over 3.3 years to prevent 1 event. A modeling study built from ASCOT-LLA later estimated a mean gain of **0.155 life-years per treated patient over a lifetime**—roughly **1.9 months**. That number must be handled carefully. It was not directly observed in the trial, and it does not mean that each prevented coronary death yielded 1.9 extra months of life. It means that when the modeled benefits are averaged across the entire population treated, including the many people who would never have suffered the event, the gain comes out to a small increment per person. Seen this way, the grandeur of the relative risk reduction gives way to something more sober: benefit that is real, but thinner, more distributed, and more dependent on baseline risk than the headline suggests. (See Kongnakorn T, Migliaccio-Walle K, Jiao T, et al. *Economic Evaluation of Atorvastatin for Prevention of Cardiovascular Events in Patients with Hypertension and Additional Risk Factors.* Value in Health. 2009. Reported mean gain: **0.155 life-years** and **0.172 QALYs** per patient over a lifetime, based on ASCOT-LLA modeling.)

In lower-risk populations (remember that ASCOT-LLA studied a high-risk population), ARR becomes even smaller. This is not an argument against statins. It is an illustration of scale. Yet when patients hear "this drug reduces your risk by 30%", many interpret this as a 30 percentage-point reduction in absolute risk, and it rarely is.

What Patients Actually Consider Meaningful

The problem is not only mathematical; it is also human. When relative risk reduction is presented without its absolute context, patients may understandably imagine that the drug is doing more than it actually is. Recent preference studies suggest that when people are given clearer information, many want far larger benefits than statins usually deliver before they consider treatment worthwhile. In a 2026 *JAMA Internal Medicine* survey of adults in the United States and Japan, participants were told that statins generally reduce cardiovascular risk by about **25% relatively** and were then asked what minimum benefit would justify taking the drug. Many wanted an **absolute risk reduction of about 7.5 percentage points**, which at common baseline risks corresponds to something on the order of a **50% to 75% relative reduction**—well beyond what typical statin trials show. Even at a **10% ten-year baseline risk**, about **42%** of participants in both countries still declined statin therapy after being informed of expected benefits and burdens.

A 2021 *JAMA Network Open* study points in the same direction. After participants reviewed **personalized benefit and harm information**, only **45%** said they would definitely or probably choose statin therapy. Willingness remained **51% or less** for risk categories below **20%**, and the risk threshold had to rise to **20%** before **75%** of respondents in that group wanted treatment. Notably, among participants with higher than 10% risk, greater health literacy, numeracy, and knowledge were associated with **less** enthusiasm for statin use, not more.

These studies do not prove that patients are "bad at statistics." If anything, they suggest something more uncomfortable: once benefits are translated into terms that resemble lived reality rather than advertising language, many patients judge the tradeoff differently than experts do. The gap, then, is not merely between absolute and relative risk. It is between what trial rhetoric implies, what patients hear, and what many patients themselves would regard as a meaningful benefit. (See Luo Y, Kawakami H, Funada S, et al. Measuring Public Preferences for Statin Therapy Using the Smallest Worthwhile Difference**.** *JAMA Internal Medicine.* 2026;186(4):488–490. doi:10.1001/jamainternmed.2025.7958, and Brodney S, Valentine KD, Sepucha K, et al. Patient Preference Distribution for Use of Statin Therapy. *JAMA Network Open.* 2021.)

Meanwhile, healthcare systems (pressured by payment models imposed by CMS and other payers) often respond to such gaps not by questioning the framing, but by intensifying pressure on clinicians. The assumption is that poor uptake or poor outcomes reflect provider failure: doctors are not following the guidelines closely enough, not prescribing aggressively enough, not completing the mandated quality measures. QUEL is a useful corrective to that reflex. In this cluster-randomized primary care trial, practices caring for patients with established coronary heart disease received a data-driven collaborative quality-improvement intervention designed to improve guideline-based care. Yet at 24 months, the intervention did **not** significantly improve **unplanned cardiovascular hospitalizations, major adverse cardiovascular events, prescribing, risk-factor target achievement, or management planning**. A related process evaluation showed that practices did engage with the program—many reported improvement efforts and found the workshops and feedback reports useful—yet that organizational activity still did not translate into better patient outcomes.

The point is not that evidence is useless or that guidelines should be ignored. It is that the habitual **blame-the-provider** model is often too crude for the reality it claims to manage. Patients are not protocols. Clinical decisions are shaped by competing illnesses, treatment burden, side effects, preferences, adherence, financial constraints, fragmented care, and the ordinary limits of human life. A system that mistakes these complexities for mere physician noncompliance will keep ratcheting up surveillance and punishment while failing to improve outcomes. The problem, in other words, is not simply that clinicians deviate from the algorithm. It is that the algorithm was never the whole story to begin with.

GLP-1 CVOTs: The Same Pattern in a New Class

The same logic now appears in a newer therapeutic key. A friend and colleague recently told me about a patient she shared with a cardiologist. The patient had well-controlled hypertension, prediabetes, and had class 1 obesity, but was otherwise fairly healthy. The cardiologist repeatedly pressed her—through messages and even in the chart—that he "should be on a GLP-1" for cardiovascular risk reduction. Notably, he did not write the prescription himself but pushed her to carry both the prescription and its consequences.

That small detail captures something about the cultural force these drugs now exert. Once a therapy acquires the glow of outcome data, the pressure to prescribe can become strangely detached from proportion, context, and even ownership of the decision. The existence of benefit in a trial begins to harden into an assumption of obligation in practice. Hesitation is made to feel like negligence; to ask for nuance is made to sound as though one is resisting evidence itself.

But this is precisely where careful reading matters most. What *do* the GLP-1 cardiovascular outcomes trials actually show? In whom were benefits demonstrated, under what conditions, over what time horizon, and to what degree? How large were the absolute benefits, and how should they be weighed against baseline risk, treatment burden, cost, body-composition effects, and the tendency of these medications to migrate far beyond the populations in which they were originally studied?

Before the moral pressure of prescription overtakes the clinical question, we have to return to the trials themselves.

Meta-analyses of GLP-1 cardiovascular outcome trials show approximately:

- ~12–15% relative reduction in MACE in high-risk populations

- Absolute risk reductions often in the range of 1–3% over several years, depending on baseline risk

For a patient with established cardiovascular disease, that ARR may be clinically meaningful. For a lower-risk patient, the absolute difference may be quite modest. The hazard ratio remains the headline figure, but the clinical relevance changes with baseline risk.

Let's take a closer look at the trials.

Interpreting the GLP-1 CVOT Landscape

LEADER (liraglutide)

- High-risk T2DM population.

- Median follow-up: 3.8 years.

- Relative reduction in MACE: ~13%.

- Absolute risk reduction: 1.9%.

- NNT ≈ 53 over ~4 years.

Interpretation:

In a secondary-prevention–weighted population, the ARR approaches 2% over four years. The NNT is 53, meaning that 53 patients in the same high risk category would have to be treated for almost 4 years to prevent *one* MACE. That may be clinically meaningful for many patients, especially those with established atherosclerotic disease. However, the hazard ratio (0.87) communicates the 13% figure more urgently than the 1.9% ARR.

SUSTAIN-6 (semaglutide)

- High baseline risk cohort

- Shorter follow-up (2.1 years)

- Larger relative reduction (~26%)

- Absolute reduction 2.3%

- NNT ≈ 43 over 2 years

Important nuance→SUSTAIN-6 was smaller and shorter, and the higher relative reduction must be interpreted in the context of:

- Event numbers

- Trial size

- Confidence intervals

- Subsequent confirmatory data

The absolute difference is modest but compressed into a short time frame.

REWIND (dulaglutide)

- Broader T2DM population
- Majority without prior CVD
- Longest follow-up (5.4 years)
- Relative reduction ~12%
- Absolute reduction 1.4%
- NNT ≈ 71 over 5 years

This trial is instructive. Lower baseline risk → smaller ARR despite similar relative reduction. Same class, different population→different clinical arithmetic.

SELECT (semaglutide in obesity, no diabetes)

- Established CVD, no diabetes.
- 3.3-year follow-up.
- Relative reduction ~20%.
- Absolute reduction 1.5%.
- NNT ≈ 67 over ~3 years.

This is particularly important for obesity medicine. For patients without diabetes but with established CVD there is demonstrable cardiovascular benefit but the absolute difference remains in the 1–2% range over ~3 years. The magnitude is real but not dramatic. It may be clinically consequential in very high-risk populations.

Table 10.2 — GLP-1 Cardiovascular Outcome Trials: Relative vs Absolute Reduction in MACE

Trial	Population (high level)	Follow-up	MACE: Drug	MACE: Placebo	Relative ↓	Absolute ↓	Approx. NNT*
LEADER	T2DM + high CV risk	3.8 y	13.0%	14.9%	13%	1.9%	~53
SUSTAIN-6	T2DM, ~83% with CVD/CKD	2.1 y	6.6%	8.9%	26%	2.3%	~44
REWIND	T2DM, mostly without prior CVD	5.4 y	12.0%	13.4%	12%	1.4%	~71
SELECT	Obesity + established CVD, no diabetes	3.3 y	6.5%	8.0%	20%	1.5%	~67

What This Table Teaches

1. Relative reductions range from 12–26%.
2. Absolute reductions cluster between 1.4–2.3%.
3. NNT ranges from ~40 to ~70 over the study duration.
4. Baseline risk drives absolute impact.
5. Follow-up duration matters.

These drugs do reduce events. However the magnitude of benefit must be interpreted in absolute terms, within a defined time horizon, and weighed against long-term physiologic trade-offs not captured in the trial endpoints.

Why This Matters for Long-Term Therapy

Relative risk reduction feels dramatic while absolute risk reduction determines NNT, cost-effectiveness, side-effect trade-offs, and patient preference alignment. When therapy is

- Lifelong

- Expensive

- Associated with body composition changes

- Potentially influencing muscle and bone over decades

then small absolute benefits may be acceptable for some patients and not for others. This is where our clinical judgement comes in.

Practical Reading Discipline for Clinicians

When reading any outcome trial:

1. Extract baseline event rate in the control group
2. Calculate or locate absolute risk reduction
3. Compute NNT for the study duration
4. Adjust mentally for your patient's baseline risk (higher or lower than trial population)
5. Consider competing risks (age, frailty, comorbid illness)

Only then does the hazard ratio acquire clinical meaning.

Anabolic Resistance, Lean Mass, and the Time Horizon Trials Do Not Capture

Anabolic resistance refers to the blunted skeletal muscle protein synthetic response to dietary protein intake, resistance exercise, and insulin signaling. This phenomenon has been demonstrated in multiple human metabolic studies using tracer methodologies. With aging:

- Higher doses of protein are required to stimulate comparable muscle protein synthesis

- Physical inactivity worsens the response

- Insulin resistance further impairs anabolic signaling

- Chronic inflammation contributes to impaired muscle remodeling

The concept is well established in gerontology and muscle physiology literature. Importantly, anabolic resistance is progressive and cumulative, starting as early as the mid 30s in sedentary individuals.

Lean Mass Loss in GLP-1 Weight Loss Trials

In major obesity trials of semaglutide (e.g., STEP program), total weight loss is substantial, and fat mass decreases significantly along with lean mass. In STEP 1, approximately 39–40% of total weight lost was lean mass by DXA. A 2026 review in the Annals of Internal Medicine by Batsis et al revealed that 68% of patients on GLP-1 medications exceeded the expected 25% muscle loss from general weight loss.

Although the *proportion* of lean mass relative to body weight may rise (because fat mass decreases more), the **absolute lean mass declines**. This distinction is often misunderstood. Absolute lean mass is what determines strength, glucose disposal capacity, functional reserve and stress tolerance.

The same pattern of meaningful fat loss accompanied by measurable lean mass loss is seen in other pharmacologic and surgical weight-loss interventions as it is a known feature of substantial negative energy balance.

Lean Mass, Glucose Disposal, and Metabolic Resilience

Skeletal muscle is the primary site of postprandial glucose disposal. Reduced muscle mass is associated with higher insulin resistance, greater glycemic variability, increased risk of type 2 diabetes progression, and higher all-cause mortality in multiple cohort studies. Although the 2026 Batsis review found no direct link between GLP-1 muscle loss and declines in strength or physical function, decreased mass alone means a smaller reservoir for glucose disposal and thus, a decline in metabolic resilience.

Sarcopenia and low appendicular lean mass have repeatedly been linked to increased hospitalization, increased mortality, and worse outcomes after surgery and infection. These associations are robust across populations.

The Long-Horizon Question

Here is where the trials become silent. We have:

- 2–5 year CVOT data

- ~1–2 year body composition data

- No randomized 10–20 year data on chronic GLP-1 use and muscle trajectories

The clinical concern crystallizes in the not-too-uncommon scenario of an aging patient on long-term GLP-1 therapy with sustained appetite suppression and inadequate protein intake and resistance training. In the context of age-related anabolic resistance with a pharmacologically sustained negative energy balance, progressive lean mass loss could accelerate transition towards a sarcopenic, or worse, a cachectic phenotype.

Frailty as the Converging Endpoint

Frailty is operationalized through gait speed, grip strength, exhaustion, weight loss, and activity measures. It is one of the strongest predictors of:

- All-cause mortality

- Cardiovascular mortality

- Hospitalization

- Institutionalization

Low muscle mass and strength are central components of frailty phenotypes. If weight-centric therapy does not explicitly preserve muscle and function, we risk shifting patients from having obesity with functional reserve to being leaner but more frail. This trade-off has not been systematically evaluated in GLP-1 outcome programs.

Clinical Implication

If GLP-1 therapy is used long term, muscle preservation must become a co-primary endpoint. Since the drug trials do not measure frailty conversion, physicians should consider baseline and follow-up body composition when feasible. (Although not covered by insurance, it is worth discussing self pay options with the patient for long-term health considerations).

Resistance training and protein dosing need to be prescribed and assessed, and not left to vague lifestyle advice. Functional measures such as gait speed and grip strength should be serially recorded. Importantly, a clear exit strategy should be delineated before starting GLP-1 therapy to outline the lean mass critical thresholds that would necessitate deprescribing.

Metabolic Paradox of Long-Term Negative Energy Balance

Short-term metabolic improvement with weight loss is real with robust data to support it. For 2–5 years, metabolic markers improve. However, weight is a composite of fat mass and lean mass (muscle, organ tissue, connective tissue, water) and GLP-1–associated weight loss includes measurable lean mass reduction. Aging independently reduces lean mass. Anabolic resistance reduces the ability to rebuild it. Yet in most clinical settings, we measure weight/BMI, A1c, and lipids, but not body composition. If A1c improves and weight decreases, we declare success. **But the primary site of insulin-mediated glucose disposal, muscle mass, is rarely tracked.**

The Physiologic Tension

As mentioned above, skeletal muscle accounts for the majority of postprandial glucose uptake. It is a determinant of insulin sensitivity and serves as a metabolic buffer during stress (infection, trauma, surgery). Reduced lean mass is associated with higher insulin resistance, increased risk of incident diabetes, and increased mortality across multiple cohorts.

So here is the paradox. We may initiate GLP-1 therapy to improve metabolic health in patients with type 2 diabetes and obesity. Short-term, weight and A1C levels decrease. But if, over 10–20 years lean mass and functional reserve decline progressively with worsening age-related anabolic resistance topped by a sustained negative energy balance, then metabolic resilience may deteriorate even if body weight remains lower than baseline.

In other words, glycemic control on a suppressed intake background does not necessarily equal preserved metabolic capacity. Those are two different constructs. We started with a patient who had diabetes and obesity and ended with diabetes and sarcopenia/frailty in the same patient. Did we actually make the patient healthier?

The Unmeasured Outcome

Current outcome trials do not answer:

- What happens to appendicular lean mass over 10–15 years?

- Does long-term GLP-1 exposure accelerate sarcopenia relative to matched controls?

- What happens to infection mortality?

- What happens to surgery/chemotherapy/hospitalization tolerance?

- What happens to fracture rates beyond initial time frames?

- What happens when these patients reach age 75–85?

We do not have those data and absence of evidence is not proof of harm nor neutrality. The assumption that weight loss equals metabolic health is empirically supported in the short term. However, it is untested across decades when lean mass becomes progressively limiting.

The Risk of Substituting One Dysfunction for Another

As we saw in the example above, it is biologically possible that **obesity-driven metabolic dysfunction may, in some individuals, be replaced over time by sarcopenia-driven metabolic vulnerability**.

Muscle loss reduces:

- Glucose disposal capacity
- Amino acid reserve
- Immune competence
- Stress tolerance

Frailty is a stronger predictor of mortality than BMI in older adults. Yet our therapeutic lens remains weight-centric. If we do not measure lean mass, we cannot detect the shift, and when late-life metabolic decline appears, we may attribute it to "genetics", "age", and/or "progression of disease" rather than to cumulative body composition changes we never tracked.

This Is Not Anti-GLP-1

It is anti-simplistic thinking. GLP-1 therapy may improve outcomes in many high-risk patients, but short-term improvements in biomarkers do not exempt us from asking what the long-term physiologic trade-offs are. Until body composition and functional endpoints are incorporated into long-horizon trials, these questions remain open.

Frailty, Sarcopenia, and Mortality: When "Lighter" Is Not the Same as "Healthier"

This section grounds the anabolic-resistance discussion in outcomes that are already well established in the literature. We are looking at survival, and not merely speculating about physiology.

Frailty as a Mortality Signal

Frailty is one of the strongest predictors of:

- All-cause mortality
- Cardiovascular mortality

- Hospitalization

- Institutionalization

Multiple meta-analyses show that individuals classified as frail have approximately 2–3× higher mortality risk compared to robust counterparts, even after adjusting for comorbidities. Frailty indices typically incorporate:

- Unintentional weight loss

- Weakness (grip strength)

- Slow gait speed

- Low physical activity

- Exhaustion

Muscle mass and muscle function are central components of this phenotype. Importantly, frailty predicts mortality independently of BMI. A person may be free of obesity and also frail. We are all well aware that BMI does not capture this risk.

Sarcopenia and Adverse Outcomes

Low appendicular lean mass and sarcopenia are associated with increased all-cause mortality (including cardiovascular mortality), worse ICU survival, and increased postoperative complications. Such patients also have higher infection-related mortality and increased fracture risk. These associations are consistent across community-dwelling older adults, hospitalized populations, dialysis patients, and oncology cohorts. We can regard low muscle mass as prognostic.

Skeletal muscle is not just structural but also the primary site of insulin-mediated glucose disposal and a reservoir of amino acids during catabolic stress. It is a regulator of systemic inflammation via myokine signaling and a determinant of basal metabolic rate. As such, loss of muscle mass reduces glucose buffering capacity, protein reserve during illness, and functional independence. **In aging populations, preservation of muscle mass and strength is more predictive of survival than reduction in body weight alone.**

The BMI/Weight Problem

We are living through a transitional moment in medicine. While we increasingly acknowledge that body composition is more clinically relevant than BMI, most pharmacologic obesity trials still use weight and BMI as primary markers of success. This creates the paradox of publicly recognizing the importance of muscle while therapeutically rewarding weight reduction without systematically measuring tissue composition.

In older adults, the so-called **obesity paradox** (where **modestly higher BMI associates with lower mortality**) may partially reflect preserved lean mass. When weight loss occurs without muscle preservation, mortality risk can rise. We see this in geriatric populations, post-hospitalization cohorts, and chronic disease states (e.g. heart failure).

Unintentional weight loss in older adults is a red flag and intentional weight loss without muscle preservation may not be benign either. The GLP-1 outcome trials were not designed to detect end-points such as frailty conversion, muscle function, and bone density. Thus we have limited data for long-term functional resilience.

So theoretically, for a 55-year-old patient with DM2 and established CVD, a 1.5–2% absolute reduction in MACE over 3–5 years may be meaningful. But if lean mass declines progressively over 15 years, and frailty risk increases as resilience to infection or surgery declines, then the long-term net effect becomes complex.

As a patient ages into their 60s and beyond, the dominant mortality risks shift toward:

- Frailty-related complications
- Falls and fractures
- Sepsis

- Functional decline

- Multimorbidity

Cardiovascular risk remains important, but muscle and function increasingly dominate survival. If our therapeutic strategy reduces cardiovascular risk modestly but erodes muscle reserve over decades, we must keep asking *what is the net effect?*

Rethinking Hunger: Hedonic, Homeostatic, and Hidden Signals

In an earlier chapter, we framed hunger in two broad categories:

1. **Homeostatic hunger** — driven by energy needs and metabolic signals.
2. **Hedonic hunger** — driven by reward circuitry and food palatability.

What I'd like to look at here is whether our categorization of "hedonic" hunger fully captures what is occurring biologically, especially in metabolically compromised individuals.

The Established Framework: Homeostatic and Hedonic Circuits

Homeostatic hunger is regulated primarily in the brain by hypothalamic nuclei (ARC, PVN, VMH) and mediated by signals such as ghrelin, leptin, insulin, GLP-1 and PYY. These signals reflect energy balance and nutrient intake.

Hedonic hunger engages mesolimbic dopamine pathways and involves the nucleus accumbens, VTA, amygdala, and prefrontal cortex. It responds to palatable, energy-dense foods and can operate independently of caloric deficit

In obesity, reward circuitry responsiveness to food cues is often heightened. Executive control networks may be relatively weakened while dopaminergic signaling may be dysregulated.

GLP-1 RAs reduce food intake through slowing gastric emptying, acting on hypothalamic centers, and modulating mesolimbic reward pathways. The appetite suppression is both metabolic and neurobehavioral.

Brain Perfusion in Obesity

Multiple imaging studies demonstrate that higher BMI is associated with reduced global and regional cerebral perfusion. Obesity correlates with reduced cerebral blood flow in frontal and temporal regions and insulin dysfunction in the brain is associated with altered cerebral glucose metabolism.

These findings are observational but consistent. Reduced brain perfusion implies reduced substrate delivery, altered metabolic demand–supply balance with potential vulnerability in executive and reward circuits.

Obesity and Brain Volume: Structural Change Beyond Perfusion

Independent of perfusion findings, a substantial neuroimaging literature demonstrates that higher BMI and metabolic dysfunction are associated with structural brain differences. Cross-sectional MRI studies consistently report:

- Lower total brain volume in individuals with obesity
- Reduced gray matter volume in prefrontal cortex, hippocampus, and anterior cingulate regions
- Alterations in white matter integrity on diffusion tensor imaging

Longitudinal studies suggest:

- Higher BMI in midlife predicts greater brain atrophy over time
- Metabolic syndrome and insulin resistance are associated with accelerated gray matter loss
- Obesity correlates with increased risk of later-life cognitive decline and dementia

The mechanisms remain debated and likely multifactorial, including chronic low-grade inflammation, cerebrovascular dysfunction, insulin resistance at the neuronal and blood–brain barrier level, and lipotoxicity and altered adipokine signaling. The question then becomes whether these measurable structural brain differences in obesity are related to behavior.

Regions consistently implicated in obesity-related volume reductions, particularly the prefrontal cortex, are involved in executive control, impulse regulation, delayed gratification, and decision-making under uncertainty.

Thus, what is often labeled "poor restraint" or "hedonic excess" may be occurring in the context of altered structural and functional neurobiology. This reframes appetite dysregulation as a potential manifestation of altered brain structure and metabolic signaling over a failure of willpower.

GLP-1 receptor agonists modulate neural reward circuitry and reduce food cue reactivity. They may partially compensate for dysregulated signaling but they do not necessarily reverse structural brain changes associated with long-standing metabolic disease.

Craving as Compensatory Signal

Given that brain perfusion is reduced in obesity and glucose remains the primary cerebral fuel under standard conditions, then increased drive to eat (particularly carbohydrate-rich food) could represent, in part, a compensatory attempt to maintain cerebral substrate delivery. This is not established as a dominant mechanism but physiologically plausible. Craving may not be purely hedonic and may represent a metabolic adaptation.

Nutrient-Driven Appetite: Evidence From Animal and Human Models

A substantial experimental literature demonstrates that appetite is not regulated by calories alone.

Protein Dilution and Hyperphagia

The Protein Leverage Hypothesis (Simpson & Raubenheimer) proposes that organisms regulate food intake to achieve a target level of protein consumption. When dietary protein is diluted:

- Rodents increase total energy intake

- They overconsume carbohydrate and fat in an attempt to meet protein needs

- Total caloric intake rises despite adequate energy availability

In a large macronutrient-mapping study in mice (Solon-Biet et al., *Cell Metabolism*, 2014) low-protein diets induced hyperphagia. Mice ate more total calories when protein percentage was reduced, suggesting that macronutrient ratio, not calorie restriction alone, drove intake behavior.

Importantly, similar patterns have been demonstrated in controlled human feeding studies. When dietary protein percentage is reduced, participants increase total caloric intake, and spontaneous energy intake decreases when they get enough protein. These findings strongly support the idea that appetite is, at least in part, nutrient-regulated rather than purely energy-regulated.

Nutrient-Specific Appetites

Beyond protein it has been shown that sodium deficiency induces specific sodium-seeking behavior in animals while iron and zinc deficiency alter feeding patterns and reward circuitry. The gut contains amino acid, fatty acid, and micronutrient sensors that communicate with central appetite networks. These systems evolved to maintain nutrient homeostasis and not simply caloric balance. Thus, increased intake in certain contexts may reflect persistent signaling from unresolved nutrient targets and an attempt to correct qualitative nutrient deficiency.

Hidden Hunger in the Context of Obesity

Modern ultra-processed diets often provide excess calories with diluted protein and micronutrient density. Epidemiologic data show that individuals with obesity frequently exhibit:

- Iron deficiency

- Vitamin D deficiency

- Magnesium deficiency

- Suboptimal protein intake relative to lean mass needs

This coexistence of caloric excess and nutrient deficiency is referred to as the **double burden of obesity**. In this context, persistent hunger may not be solely "hedonic." It may represent:

- Incomplete nutrient satisfaction

- Protein-driven intake compensation

- Micronutrient-seeking behavior masked by caloric abundance

This does not eliminate the role of reward circuitry. It suggests that reward amplification may coexist with unresolved nutrient signaling.

Implications for GLP-1–Mediated Appetite Suppression

GLP-1 receptor agonists suppress appetite broadly. They do not distinguish between excess caloric intake, protein-seeking intake, micronutrient-driven intake, and reward-driven intake. If dietary quality is not simultaneously improved, pharmacologic appetite suppression may reduce protein intake while failing to correct micronutrient deficiencies. This biologically plausible concern is grounded in established nutrient-regulation science and may contribute to worsening anabolic resistance over time.

Reframing Hedonic Hunger

If obesity involves:

- Structural brain differences
- Altered reward circuitry
- Nutrient dilution
- Protein leverage dynamics
- Micronutrient deficiencies
- Insulin resistance

then labeling all excess intake as "hedonic hunger" may be reductive. Some hunger may be metabolic, structural, and/or compensatory. If we conceptualize all hunger in obesity as "hedonic excess," we default to suppression as the solution. When we acknowledge that some hunger may reflect

- Impaired perfusion
- Insulin resistance
- Nutrient dilution
- Protein leverage
- Micronutrient deficit

appetite suppression alone may not fully resolve underlying metabolic drivers. In long-term GLP-1 therapy, this raises critical questions

- Are we correcting metabolic dysfunction?
- Or are we suppressing signals arising from it?
- Does nutrient quality become more important, not less, under pharmacologic suppression?

Layering GLP-1 Signaling: Surgery, Pharmacology, and the Central Axis

GLP-1 receptor agonists and bariatric surgery are often treated as separate therapeutic pathways. Increasingly, they are intersecting in clinical care. To understand what that means physiologically, we must distinguish:

- Peripheral GLP-1 secretion
- Central GLP-1 production
- Pharmacologic receptor stimulation

After Roux-en-Y gastric bypass (RYGB), and to a lesser extent sleeve gastrectomy, postprandial GLP-1 secretion increases markedly. Mechanistically, surgery accelerates nutrient delivery to the distal intestine. It increases L-cell stimulation, alters bile acid signaling and modifies vagal afferent input. The GLP-1 rise is nutrient-triggered and pulsatile and fasting levels are not chronically elevated. Exaggerated GLP-1 responses contribute to improved insulin secretion and glycemia to the extent that in some cases, excessive postprandial GLP-1 contributes to hypoglycemia. Importantly, surgery amplifies meal-dependent GLP-1 spikes and not continuous receptor stimulation.

GLP-1 is also produced centrally by preproglucagon neurons in the nucleus tractus solitarius (NTS), projecting widely to the hypothalamus, amygdala, and other appetite and stress centers in the brain. Visceral sensory input, gastric distension, nutrient signaling, aversive stimuli, and stress activate central GLP-1 neurons. This system integrates satiety, stress responses, nausea and reward modulation.

Peripheral GLP-1 does not freely cross the blood–brain barrier in significant amounts. Endogenous central GLP-1 is locally regulated. Thus bariatric surgery amplifies peripheral GLP-1 spikes, which signal through vagal and circumventricular pathways, but central GLP-1 production remains physiologically regulated.

Clinically, GLP-1 RAs are used after bariatric surgery for weight regain or insufficient response. Short-term studies show additional weight loss and glycemic improvement and safety appears broadly consistent. However these studies are short duration, body composition is rarely central, and functional outcomes are not tracked.

When combining exaggerated postprandial peripheral GLP-1 spikes (surgery) with sustained pharmacologic receptor activation (GLP-1 RA), we create a signaling environment that is not physiologic. We do not have long-horizon neuro-metabolic outcome data and many questions remain unanswered:

- Does chronic receptor stimulation alter central GLP-1 neuron activity?

- Does long-term modulation of mesolimbic circuits affect reward regulation beyond appetite?

- Does sustained central signaling influence stress responses or immune tone?

- Does appetite suppression layered on altered anatomy affect protein and micronutrient sufficiency over decades?

Bariatric surgery alone is associated with lean mass reduction, decreased bone mineral density, increased fracture risk over long-term follow-up, and micronutrient deficiencies. GLP-1 RAs independently reduce lean mass in proportion to total weight loss. Thus, layering these therapies raises legitimate questions:

- Is sarcopenia risk amplified?

- Is bone loss compounded?

- Does sustained appetite suppression exacerbate protein insufficiency?

- What are frailty trajectories 15–20 years later?

Trophic Concerns

Some studies show that L-cells express the GLP-1 receptor. L-cell function or survival might then be modulated through feed-forward or feedback loops by exogenous agonists. After Roux-en-Y surgery there is increased endogenous GLP-1 production. Adding GLP-1 medications may stimulate potent growth signals in the intestinal lining.

GLP-1 promotes crypt fission, leading to an increase in the width and length of the small and large bowel and animal studies show the increase in mucosal surface as well. These effects are generally accepted as being protective but some studies have shown that in specific genetic models of intestinal cancer, crypt fission has increased the number and size of polyps through GLP-1 receptor activation. We have seen this in animal models and human registry studies have not confirmed this at the current time.

There is mixed and controversial data regarding Roux-en-Y gastric bypass (RYGB) and colorectal cancer. A very large 2023 meta-analysis showed protection in people with morbid obesity who underwent the surgery but several long follow-up cohort studies have shown increased risk for those who were greater than ten years out from their surgery. Some retrospective studies have shown more precancerous polyps five or more years after RYGB.

Given this complex and conflicting data, adding pharmacologic GLP-1 agents needs to be decided with caution. There should be a higher suspicion index with new and unusual symptoms, and consideration of more frequent screening ten or more years after surgery.

The question is whether long-term functional reserve is being preserved with combined therapy. GLP-1 signaling is not a single pathway. It is:

- Peripheral endocrine
- Central neuroregulatory
- Integrated with stress, inflammation, and reward circuits

When we pharmacologically sustain a system designed for pulsatile activation and layer that on surgically altered anatomy, we enter territory not fully characterized by current outcome trials.

From Following Guidelines to Practicing Judgment

Modern medicine is saturated with guidelines, algorithms, risk calculators, meta-analyses, and AI-generated summaries. While these are valuable tools, they operate at the level of population averages and predefined endpoints. They should not constitute the practice of medicine.

Guidelines synthesize relative risk reductions, hazard ratios, predefined composite endpoints, and short-to-intermediate follow-up durations. They clearly reflect only the endpoints that were measured. While they provide treatment thresholds, risk-based stratification, and class I/II/III recommendations, there are a number of factors they do not incorporate well such as

- Long-term body composition trajectories
- Frailty conversion
- Functional reserve
- Nutrient adequacy
- Brain structural change
- Patient-specific tolerance for modest absolute benefit

Every field and industry sector has been plagued by the question of whether people can be replaced by AI, and medicine is no exception. It has become increasingly obvious that AI exceeds human capacity in certain respects. An AI system can:

- Extract hazard ratios
- Calculate absolute risk reduction

- Compute NNT
- Summarize guideline recommendations
- Compare meta-analyses

In other words, AI can perform evidence parsing faster than any physician. So if our role as physicians is limited to applying guidelines to risk scores, we are inarguably replaceable, and sooner than we think.

What cannot be automated is the integration of:

- Competing risks across decades
- Short-term cardiovascular benefit versus long-term frailty risk
- Absolute risk reduction versus patient value thresholds
- Body composition shifts versus metabolic biomarkers
- Appetite suppression versus nutrient adequacy
- Structural brain change versus behavioral interpretation

Judgment requires temporal reasoning, the weighing of trade-offs, uncertainty tolerance. Most of all, it requires legal accountability and moral responsibility. And this means asking the hard questions that trials do not touch.

Moving Beyond Weight-Centric Medicine (Please!)

We publicly acknowledge that body composition matters more than BMI and still, we chase that number on the scale or the A1C and non-specific inflammatory markers. But the full spectrum of metabolic health includes muscle mass, functional strength, immune competence, bone integrity, resilience, and cognitive stability. All of these outcomes emerge over decades and are rarely primary endpoints in studies.

Our role as physicians is neither to defend drugs nor to oppose them reflexively. We are called to

- Understand what was measured
- Recognize what was not
- Integrate physiology with trial arithmetic
- Align decisions with patient values
- Revisit decisions as new data emerge

Evidence informs, but it is Judgment that is needed to decide and to deliver state-of-the-art patient care. In an era of aggressive pharmaceutical marketing, simplified public narratives, and weight-centric cultural bias, that distinction becomes more important, not less.

The GLP-1 trials tell us what happens over 2–5 years. They do not tell us what happens over 15–20. In that unmeasured decade, resilience may determine survival more than BMI. Those are the years that matter most to our patients. May we not disappoint their trust in us.

Bottom Line

Understanding the difference between relative and absolute risk is essential to interpreting the true magnitude of benefit. Similarly, recognizing that weight loss includes both fat and lean mass is critical to evaluating long-term health.

As access to these medications expands, the need for thoughtful medical oversight becomes more important.

****

Reclaiming the Discipline of Medicine

This book is purportedly about GLP-1–how it works, its role in the metabolic-immune system, and the ramifications of overriding our physiology. We have moved through endocrine signaling, immune modulation, body composition, metabolic hysteresis, control theory, frailty, nutrient-driven appetite, structural brain change, and the arithmetic of risk. We have examined how trials are designed, how relative risk shapes perception, and how easily weight becomes a proxy for health. While GLP-1 receptor agonists served as the entry point, they were never the true subject. The main point and subject was **how we think**.

There is an ongoing contraction happening in medicine. We are increasingly rewarded for applying guidelines efficiently, quoting hazard ratios accurately, and optimizing biomarkers to target ranges. Physiology does not exist inside guideline tables but inside adaptive systems that trade short-term gains for long-term costs, compensate for perturbations, and carry forward the imprint of past exposures. When we reduce medicine to protocol adherence, we practice at the surface of those systems rather than within them.

Is this Enough? Is it enough to recite drug trials to colleagues and patients? Is it enough to optimize A1C and celebrate weight loss without measuring muscle? Is it enough to quote relative risk without translating absolute consequence? Is it enough to follow consensus when the endpoints themselves are narrow?

If medicine becomes mere regurgitation of published conclusions, then we have mistaken information for understanding and confused repetition with judgment. At some point we, as the gatekeepers of our patients' safety and care, must also say Enough.

Enough of fragmented care that isolates organs from systems. Enough of siloed thinking that separates metabolism from immunity, muscle from glucose, brain from behavior. Enough of simplistic models that equate weight with health and suppression with solution. Enough of pretending that what is unmeasured is irrelevant.

Medical education must evolve accordingly. It must teach systems science alongside pharmacology, control theory alongside endocrinology, absolute risk alongside relative risk, and functional preservation alongside disease suppression. It must train physicians to see trade-offs, tolerate uncertainty, and think temporally. Without that depth, we risk becoming technicians of consensus rather than stewards of physiology.

This is not a rejection of pharmacology. It is a refusal to let pharmacology define the entirety of care. GLP-1 was the case study. The deeper lesson is that medicine is the care of complex living systems over time. It requires integration, discernment, and the courage to acknowledge what is unknown.

Enough, then, is not about scarcity. It is about sufficiency of thought. Are we thinking deeply enough? Measuring comprehensively enough? Teaching broadly enough? Caring longitudinally enough?

The future of healthcare should not rest in repeating data, however efficiently and earnestly. It demands systems integration and the application of first principles in problem solving. If we wish to remain essential and not merely operational, we must reclaim this discipline of critical thinking by measuring what truly matters, and practicing with judgment that extends beyond the duration of any trial.

The question is not whether any drug, GLP-1 RA or otherwise, is enough. The question is whether the way we practice is.

Epilogue

Summer was sodden with scorch and blaze. By the time Ed arrived, the city was drowsy and dazed with heat stroke. The movers had come and gone but there were still piles to be sorted and disposed of. My workout tower for pullups and dips was too big for me to tackle alone. There was the bench and the weights I had been too tired to haul to Goodwill, along with random kitchen utensils, appliances and electronics. He took one look at the scattered piles and started posting things online for free takeaway.

We rented a van for everything to be donated: the bags of winter clothes I wouldn't need again, bins of Tom's clothing now freed from memory, strange gadgets and leftover tools from M's days, boxes of orphan dongles, cords and plugs, and dinosaur electronic devices long obsolete. In the car were my suitcases, paintings, one box of books, and Tula's ashes. People came in and out to cart away the workout equipment. Ed took me to Andala Cafe for my favourite omelette. We even had Malaysian food at Penang for lunch, one last taste of *assam ikan bilis* and *kangkung belacan* before I said goodbye.

And then we were driving, last merge off the ramp onto the Mass Pike, Ed at the wheel while I took in my final views of Boston. We would drive for days, through fog, rain, flood and a flat battery towards a new start. In an evening gold with promise, I saw his profile steady and reassuring against a flickering world. After all these years he had flown across the country to move me once again.

The land opened up and we were *following the river down the highway through the cradle of the Civil War*. That drone again, the chug of the guitar. The miles piled behind us like shed lives. After losses and losses, love and hope again, and *I've reason to believe we both will be received in Graceland.*

Core References

Chapter 1

Bode, J. G., Albrecht, U., Häussinger, D., Heinrich, P. C., & Schaper, F. (2012). Hepatic acute phase proteins—Regulation by IL-6- and IL-1-type cytokines involving STAT3 and its crosstalk with NF-κB-dependent signaling. *European Journal of Cell Biology, 91*(6–7), 496–505.

Re: IL-6 and IL-1 regulation of hepatic acute-phase protein production.

Dantzer, R., O'Connor, J. C., Freund, G. G., Johnson, R. W., & Kelley, K. W. (2008). From inflammation to sickness and depression: When the immune system subjugates the brain. *Nature Reviews Neuroscience, 9*(1), 46–56.

Re: Sickness behavior, fatigue, appetite change, social withdrawal, and brain–immune signaling.

DeLany, J. P., Kelley, D. E., Hames, K. C., Jakicic, J. M., & Goodpaster, B. H. (2013). High energy expenditure masks low physical activity in obesity. *International Journal of Obesity, 37*(7), 1006–1011.

Re: Higher energy expenditure in obesity, especially as related to greater body mass and fat-free mass.

Furman, D., Campisi, J., Verdin, E., Carrera-Bastos, P., Targ, S., Franceschi, C., Ferrucci, L., Gilroy, D. W., Fasano, A., Miller, G. W., et al. (2019). Chronic inflammation in the etiology of disease across the life span. *Nature Medicine, 25*, 1822–1832.

Re: Chronic inflammation as a biological driver across multiple diseases and across the lifespan.

Hu, T., Liu, C.-H., Lei, M., Zeng, Q., Li, L., Tang, H., & Zhang, N. (2024). Metabolic regulation of the immune system in health and diseases: Mechanisms and interventions. *Signal Transduction and Targeted Therapy, 9*, 268.

Re: Immunometabolism; how metabolic pathways regulate immune-cell behavior.

Jeschke, M. G., Chinkes, D. L., Finnerty, C. C., Kulp, G., Suman, O. E., Norbury, W. B., Branski, L. K., Gauglitz, G. G., & Herndon, D. N. (2008). Pathophysiologic response to severe burn injury. *Annals of Surgery, 248*(3), 387–401.

Re: Severe inflammation, hypermetabolism, and catabolism after major burn injury.

Jeschke, M. G., Gauglitz, G. G., Kulp, G. A., Finnerty, C. C., Williams, F. N., Kraft, R., Suman, O. E., Mlcak, R. P., & Herndon, D. N. (2011). Long-term persistence of the pathophysiologic response to severe burn injury. *PLOS ONE, 6*(7), e21245.

Re: Prolonged hypermetabolic and catabolic response after severe burn injury.

Kistner, T. M., Pedersen, B. K., & Lieberman, D. E. (2022). Interleukin 6 as an energy allocator in muscle tissue. *Nature Metabolism, 4*, 170–179.

Re: IL-6 as an energy allocation signal, especially in skeletal muscle and exercise physiology.

Mantovani, A., Garlanda, C., Doni, A., & Bottazzi, B. (2023). Humoral innate immunity and acute-phase proteins. *New England Journal of Medicine, 388*, 439–452.

Re: Acute-phase proteins as part of innate immune defense.

Pedersen, B. K., & Febbraio, M. A. (2008). Muscle as an endocrine organ: Focus on muscle-derived interleukin-6. *Physiological Reviews, 88*(4), 1379–1406.

Re: Skeletal muscle as an endocrine organ; exercise-induced IL-6 as a myokine.

Rall, L. C., & Roubenoff, R. (2004). Rheumatoid cachexia: Metabolic abnormalities, mechanisms and interventions. *Rheumatology, 43*(10), 1219–1223.

Re: Chronic inflammation, increased resting energy expenditure, and protein catabolism in rheumatoid cachexia.

Roubenoff, R., Roubenoff, R. A., Cannon, J. G., Kehayias, J. J., Zhuang, H., Dawson-Hughes, B., Dinarello, C. A., & Rosenberg, I. H. (1994). Rheumatoid cachexia: Cytokine-driven hypermetabolism accompanying reduced body cell mass in chronic inflammation. *Journal of Clinical Investigation, 93*(6), 2379–2386.

Re: Cytokine-associated hypermetabolism and reduced body cell mass in chronic inflammatory disease.

Straub, R. H., Cutolo, M., Buttgereit, F., & Pongratz, G. (2010). Energy regulation and neuroendocrine–immune control in chronic inflammatory diseases. *Journal of Internal Medicine, 267*(6), 543–560.

Re: Energy regulation, fuel allocation, and neuroendocrine–immune control in chronic inflammatory disease.

Straub, R. H. (2012). Evolutionary medicine and chronic inflammatory state—Known and new concepts in pathophysiology. *Journal of Molecular Medicine, 90*, 523–534.

Re: Chronic inflammatory states as energy-demanding conditions involving fuel redistribution.

Zatterale, F., Longo, M., Naderi, J., Raciti, G. A., Desiderio, A., Miele, C., & Beguinot, F. (2020). Chronic adipose tissue inflammation linking obesity to insulin resistance and type 2 diabetes. *Frontiers in Physiology, 10*, 1607.

Re: Adipose tissue inflammation, obesity, insulin resistance, and type 2 diabetes.

Chapter 2

Albrechtsen, N. J. W., Junker, A. E., Christensen, M., Hædersdal, S., Wibrand, F., Lund, A. M., Galsgaard, K. D., Holst, J. J., & Knop, F. K. (2019). The liver–α-cell axis and type 2 diabetes. *Endocrine Reviews, 40*(5), 1353–1366.

Re: The liver–alpha cell axis; glucagon, amino acid clearance, ureagenesis, hepatic steatosis, and type 2 diabetes.

Alhadeff, A. L., Rupprecht, L. E., & Hayes, M. R. (2012). GLP-1 neurons in the nucleus of the solitary tract project directly to the ventral tegmental area and nucleus accumbens to control for food intake. *Endocrinology, 153*(2), 647–658.

Re: Central GLP-1 neurons projecting from the NTS to reward-related regions involved in food intake.

Bell, G. I., Santerre, R. F., & Mullenbach, G. T. (1983). Hamster preproglucagon contains the sequence of glucagon and two related peptides. *Nature, 302,* 716–718.

Re: Discovery that proglucagon contains glucagon and glucagon-like peptide sequences within a larger precursor molecule.

Bell, G. I., Sanchez-Pescador, R., Laybourn, P. J., & Najarian, R. C. (1983). Exon duplication and divergence in the human preproglucagon gene. *Nature, 304,* 368–371.

Re: Human preproglucagon gene structure and the molecular lineage of glucagon-related peptides.

Drucker, D. J. (2005). Biologic actions and therapeutic potential of the proglucagon-derived peptides. *Nature Clinical Practice Endocrinology & Metabolism, 1,* 22–31.

Re: Proglucagon-derived peptides as a coordinated hormonal family, including glucagon, GLP-1, GLP-2, and oxyntomodulin.

Drucker, D. J. (2018). Mechanisms of action and therapeutic application of glucagon-like peptide-1. *Cell Metabolism, 27*(4), 740–756.

Re: GLP-1 physiology, pharmacology, incretin action, appetite effects, and therapeutic GLP-1 receptor agonists.

Eng, J., Kleinman, W. A., Singh, L., Singh, G., & Raufman, J.-P. (1992). Isolation and characterization of exendin-4, an exendin-3 analogue, from *Heloderma suspectum* venom. *Journal of Biological Chemistry, 267*(11), 7402–7405.

Re: Discovery of exendin-4 from Gila monster venom, the peptide that led to exenatide.

Gasbjerg, L. S., Helsted, M. M., Hartmann, B., Jensen, M. H., Gabe, M. B. N., Sparre-Ulrich, A. H., Veedfald, S., Stensen, S., Lanng, A. R., Bergmann, N. C., Christensen, M. B., Vilsbøll, T., Holst, J. J., Rosenkilde, M. M., & Knop, F. K. (2019). Separate and combined glucometabolic effects of endogenous glucose-dependent insulinotropic polypeptide and glucagon-like peptide-1 in healthy individuals. *Diabetes, 68*(5), 906–917.

Re: Coordinated and distinct roles of GIP and GLP-1 in postprandial glucose metabolism.

Holst, J. J. (2007). The physiology of glucagon-like peptide-1. *Physiological Reviews, 87*(4), 1409–1439.

Re: Foundational GLP-1 physiology, secretion, degradation, incretin effects, glucagon suppression, gastric emptying, and appetite.

Holst, J. J. (2019). The incretin system in healthy humans: The role of GIP and GLP-1. *Metabolism, 96*, 46–55.

Re: Human incretin physiology and the complementary roles of GIP and GLP-1.

Kimball, C. P., & Murlin, J. R. (1923). Aqueous extracts of pancreas. III. Some precipitation reactions of insulin. *Journal of Biological Chemistry, 58*, 337–346.

Re: Early identification of a pancreatic hyperglycemic factor later named glucagon.

Müller, T. D., Finan, B., Clemmensen, C., DiMarchi, R. D., & Tschöp, M. H. (2017). The new biology and pharmacology of glucagon. *Physiological Reviews, 97*(2), 721–766.

Re: Modern glucagon physiology, including glucose regulation, amino acid metabolism, and therapeutic implications.

Nauck, M. A., & Meier, J. J. (2018). Incretin hormones: Their role in health and disease. *Diabetes, Obesity and Metabolism, 20*(Suppl. 1), 5–21.

Re: GIP and GLP-1 physiology, incretin effects, type 2 diabetes, and therapeutic implications.

Novo Nordisk. (2025). *Wegovy® tablets prescribing information*. U.S. Food and Drug Administration.

Re: Oral semaglutide pharmacokinetics, steady-state concentrations, albumin binding, and extended pharmacologic exposure.

Richter, M. M., Holst, J. J., & Albrechtsen, N. J. W. (2022). The liver–α-cell axis in health and in disease. *International Journal of Molecular Sciences, 23*(23), 15248.

Re: Amino acid–glucagon feedback, hepatic amino acid metabolism, ureagenesis, and alpha-cell adaptation.

Sandoval, D. A., & D'Alessio, D. A. (2015). Physiology of proglucagon peptides: Role of glucagon and GLP-1 in health and disease. *Physiological Reviews, 95*(2), 513–548.

Re: Proglucagon biology, tissue-specific processing, glucagon, GLP-1, pancreatic islets, gut, and brain.

Secher, A., Jelsing, J., Baquero, A. F., Hecksher-Sørensen, J., Cowley, M. A., Dalbøge, L. S., Hansen, G., Grove, K. L., Pyke, C., Raun, K., Schäffer, L., Tang-Christensen, M., Verma, S., Witgen, B. M., Vrang, N., & Bjerre Knudsen, L. (2014). The arcuate nucleus mediates GLP-1 receptor agonist liraglutide-dependent weight loss. *Journal of Clinical Investigation, 124*(10), 4473–4488.

Re: Central GLP-1 receptor access and hypothalamic mechanisms of GLP-1 receptor agonist–induced weight loss.

U.S. Food and Drug Administration. (2026). *Zepbound® (tirzepatide) prescribing information*.

Re: Tirzepatide pharmacokinetics, albumin binding, half-life, and once-weekly pharmacologic exposure.

Williams, D. L. (2014). Neural integration of satiation and food reward: Role of GLP-1 and orexin pathways. *Physiology & Behavior, 136*, 194–199.

Re: GLP-1 signaling at the intersection of satiation, food reward, and motivated feeding.

Chapter 3

Albrechtsen, N. J. W., Junker, A. E., Christensen, M., Hædersdal, S., Wibrand, F., Lund, A. M., Galsgaard, K. D., Holst, J. J., & Knop, F. K. (2019). The liver–α-cell axis and type 2 diabetes. *Endocrine Reviews, 40*(5), 1353–1366.

Re: Liver–alpha-cell axis; glucagon, amino acid clearance, ureagenesis, hepatic steatosis, and type 2 diabetes.

Baggio, L. L., & Drucker, D. J. (2021). Glucagon-like peptide-1 receptor co-agonists for treating metabolic disease. *Molecular Metabolism, 46*, 101090.

Re: GLP-1 receptor co-agonists, dual/triple agonist strategies, and the therapeutic logic of multi-receptor incretin drugs.

Drucker, D. J. (2018). Mechanisms of action and therapeutic application of glucagon-like peptide-1. *Cell Metabolism, 27*(4), 740–756.

Re: GLP-1 physiology, GLP-1 receptor agonists, glucose lowering, appetite, gastric emptying, and therapeutic pharmacology.

Frías, J. P., Davies, M. J., Rosenstock, J., Pérez Manghi, F. C., Fernández Landó, L., Bergman, B. K., Liu, B., Cui, X., Brown, K., & SURPASS-2 Investigators. (2021). Tirzepatide versus semaglutide once weekly in patients with type 2 diabetes. *New England Journal of Medicine, 385*, 503–515.

Re: Tirzepatide as a dual GIP/GLP-1 receptor agonist in type 2 diabetes; glycemic and weight-loss efficacy.

Gelling, R. W., Du, X. Q., Dichmann, D. S., Romer, J., Huang, H., Cui, L., Obici, S., Tang, B., Holst, J. J., Fledelius, C., Johansen, P. B., Rossetti, L., Jelicks, L. A., Serup, P., Nishimura, E., & Charron, M. J. (2003). Lower blood glucose, hyperglucagonemia, and pancreatic α-cell hyperplasia in glucagon receptor knockout mice. *Proceedings of the National Academy of Sciences, 100*(3), 1438–1443.

Re: Glucagon receptor disruption, alpha-cell hyperplasia, hyperglucagonemia, and altered glucose/amino-acid physiology.

Holst, J. J. (2007). The physiology of glucagon-like peptide-1. *Physiological Reviews, 87*(4), 1409–1439.

Re: Foundational GLP-1 physiology, incretin effects, glucagon suppression, gastric emptying, appetite, and rapid degradation of native GLP-1.

Jastreboff, A. M., Aronne, L. J., Ahmad, N. N., Wharton, S., Connery, L., Alves, B., Kiyosue, A., Zhang, S., Liu, B., Bunck, M. C., Stefanski, A., & SURMOUNT-1 Investigators. (2022). Tirzepatide once weekly for the treatment of obesity. *New England Journal of Medicine, 387*, 205–216.

Re: Tirzepatide for chronic weight management; dual incretin agonism and magnitude of weight loss.

Jastreboff, A. M., Kaplan, L. M., Frías, J. P., Wu, Q., Du, Y., Gurbuz, S., Coskun, T., Haupt, A., Milicevic, Z., Hartman, M. L., & Retatrutide Phase 2 Obesity Trial Investigators. (2023). Triple–hormone-receptor agonist retatrutide for obesity. *New England Journal of Medicine, 389*, 514–526.

Re: Retatrutide as a GIP/GLP-1/glucagon receptor agonist; triple agonism, weight loss, and adverse effects.

Lutter, M., Bahl, E., Hannah, C., Hofammann, D., Acevedo, S., Cui, H., McAdams, C. J., & Michaelson, J. J. (2017). Novel and ultra-rare damaging variants in neuropeptide signaling are associated with disordered eating behaviors. *PLOS ONE, 12*(8), e0181556.

Re: Rare variants in neuropeptide signaling, including GLP-1/GLP-1R pathways; useful for distinguishing rare signaling defects from common "GLP-1 deficiency" claims.

Meier, J. J. (2010). Is the diminished incretin effect in type 2 diabetes just an epiphenomenon of impaired β-cell function? *Diabetes, 59*(5), 1117–1125.

Re: Impaired incretin effect in type 2 diabetes and the question of whether this reflects primary incretin failure or downstream beta-cell dysfunction.

Nauck, M. A., Vardarli, I., Deacon, C. F., Holst, J. J., & Meier, J. J. (2011). Secretion of glucagon-like peptide-1 in type 2 diabetes mellitus: Systematic review and meta-analyses of clinical studies. *Diabetologia, 54*, 10–18.

Re: GLP-1 secretion in type 2 diabetes; evidence against a simple universal GLP-1 deficiency model.

Nugraha, I. B. A., Saraswati, M. R., & Suastika, K. (2019). The pattern of fasting and post 75 g glucose loading of glucagon-like peptide 1 levels in obese and non-obese subjects. *Open Access Macedonian Journal of Medical Sciences, 7*(3), 358–362.

Re: GLP-1 levels after glucose loading in individuals with and without obesity; modest/variable differences rather than absence of GLP-1 secretion.

Nauck, M. A., Quast, D. R., Wefers, J., & Meier, J. J. (2021). GLP-1 receptor agonists in the treatment of type 2 diabetes: State-of-the-art. *Molecular Metabolism, 46*, 101102.

Re: GLP-1 receptor agonists in type 2 diabetes; pharmacologic mechanisms, glucose lowering, weight loss, and tolerability.

Nauck, M. A., & Meier, J. J. (2023). Incretin hormones and type 2 diabetes. *Diabetologia, 66*, 1780–1795.

Re: Incretin physiology, reduced incretin effect in type 2 diabetes, GLP-1/GIP actions, glucagon, appetite, and therapeutic implications.

Richter, M. M., Holst, J. J., & Albrechtsen, N. J. W. (2022). The liver–α-cell axis in health and in disease. *International Journal of Molecular Sciences, 23*(23), 15248.

Re: Amino acid–glucagon feedback, hepatic amino-acid metabolism, ureagenesis, alpha-cell adaptation, and disease states.

U.S. Food and Drug Administration. (2026). *Zepbound® (tirzepatide) prescribing information.*

Re: Tirzepatide pharmacokinetics, albumin binding, half-life, dosing, and safety labeling.

Winther-Sørensen, M., Galsgaard, K. D., Santos, A., Trammell, S. A. J., Sulek, K., Kuhre, R. E., Pedersen, J., Andersen, D. B., Hassing, A. S., Dall, M., Treebak, J. T., Gillum, M. P., Wewer Albrechtsen, N. J., & Holst, J. J. (2020). Glucagon acutely regulates hepatic amino acid catabolism and the effect may be disturbed by steatosis. *Molecular Metabolism, 42*, 101080.

Re: Glucagon regulation of hepatic amino-acid catabolism, ureagenesis, and disruption by hepatic steatosis.

Chapter 4

Atherton, P. J., & Smith, K. (2012). Muscle protein synthesis in response to nutrition and exercise. *Journal of Physiology, 590*(5), 1049–1057.

Re: Muscle protein synthesis, amino acid availability, resistance exercise, and anabolic signaling.

Bauer, J., Biolo, G., Cederholm, T., Cesari, M., Cruz-Jentoft, A. J., Morley, J. E., Phillips, S., Sieber, C., Stehle, P., Teta, D., Visvanathan, R., Volpi, E., & Boirie, Y. (2013). Evidence-based recommendations for optimal dietary protein intake in older people: A position paper from the PROT-AGE Study Group. *Journal of the American Medical Directors Association, 14*(8), 542–559.

Re: Protein intake, aging muscle, anabolic resistance, and the need for higher-quality protein distribution in vulnerable adults.

Breen, L., & Phillips, S. M. (2011). Skeletal muscle protein metabolism in the elderly: Interventions to counteract the "anabolic resistance" of ageing. *Nutrition & Metabolism, 8*, 68.

Re: Anabolic resistance, aging muscle, protein stimulation, and resistance training.

Dulloo, A. G., Jacquet, J., & Girardier, L. (1997). Poststarvation hyperphagia and body fat overshooting in humans: A role for feedback signals from lean and fat tissues. *American Journal of Clinical Nutrition, 65*(3), 717–723.

Re: Preferential fat regain after weight loss, lean tissue recovery, and "fat overshooting."

Guillet, C., Prod'homme, M., Balage, M., Gachon, P., Giraudet, C., Morin, L., Grizard, J., & Boirie, Y. (2004). Impaired anabolic response of muscle protein synthesis is associated with S6K1 dysregulation in elderly humans. *FASEB Journal, 18*(13), 1586–1587.

Re: Muscle anabolic resistance and impaired mTOR/S6K1 signaling with aging.

Heymsfield, S. B., Gonzalez, M. C., Shen, W., Redman, L., & Thomas, D. (2014). Weight loss composition is one-fourth fat-free mass: A critical review and critique of this widely cited rule. *Obesity Reviews, 15*(4), 310–321.

Re: Composition of weight loss, fat mass vs fat-free mass, and why lean mass loss varies by context.

Jastreboff, A. M., Aronne, L. J., Ahmad, N. N., Wharton, S., Connery, L., Alves, B., Kiyosue, A., Zhang, S., Liu, B., Bunck, M. C., Stefanski, A., & SURMOUNT-1 Investigators. (2022). Tirzepatide once weekly for the treatment of obesity. *New England Journal of Medicine, 387*, 205–216.

Re: Tirzepatide-associated weight loss in obesity; clinical context for large-magnitude pharmacologic weight reduction.

Kim, J., Wang, Z., Heymsfield, S. B., Baumgartner, R. N., & Gallagher, D. (2002). Total-body skeletal muscle mass: Estimation by a new dual-energy X-ray absorptiometry method. *American Journal of Clinical Nutrition, 76*(2), 378–383.

Re: DXA-derived estimates of skeletal muscle mass and interpretation of lean tissue compartments.

Mele, C., Mai, S., Vietti, R., Aimaretti, G., Scacchi, M., & Marzullo, P. (2022). Bone response to weight loss following bariatric surgery. *Frontiers in Endocrinology, 13*, 921353.

Re: Bone mineral density, bone turnover, mechanical unloading, and skeletal effects after major weight loss.

Moore, D. R., Robinson, M. J., Fry, J. L., Tang, J. E., Glover, E. I., Wilkinson, S. B., Prior, T., Tarnopolsky, M. A., & Phillips, S. M. (2009). Ingested protein dose response of muscle and albumin protein synthesis after resistance exercise in young men. *American Journal of Clinical Nutrition, 89*(1), 161–168.

Re: Per-meal protein dose, amino acid threshold, and muscle protein synthesis response.

Neeland, I. J., Marso, S. P., Ayers, C. R., Lewis, B., Oslica, R., Francis, W., Roddy, T., & Adams-Huet, B. (2024). Changes in lean body mass with glucagon-like peptide-1–based therapies and mitigation strategies. *Diabetes, Obesity and Metabolism, 26*(11), 4322–4331.

Re: Lean body mass changes with GLP-1-based therapies, body composition interpretation, and mitigation strategies.

Phillips, S. M. (2014). A brief review of critical processes in exercise-induced muscular hypertrophy. *Sports Medicine, 44*(Suppl. 1), S71–S77.

Re: Mechanical loading, resistance training, muscle protein synthesis, and hypertrophy.

Paddon-Jones, D., & Rasmussen, B. B. (2009). Dietary protein recommendations and the prevention of sarcopenia. *Current Opinion in Clinical Nutrition and Metabolic Care, 12*(1), 86–90.

Re: Protein distribution, meal-based protein dosing, and sarcopenia prevention.

Prado, C. M., Purcell, S. A., & Alish, C. (2018). Implications of low muscle mass across the continuum of care: A narrative review. *Annals of Medicine, 50*(8), 675–693.

Re: Clinical implications of low muscle mass, frailty, function, and outcomes.

Sartori, R., Romanello, V., & Sandri, M. (2021). Mechanisms of muscle atrophy and hypertrophy: Implications in health and disease. *Nature Communications, 12*, 330.

Re: Muscle atrophy, hypertrophy, mTOR, proteolysis, nutrient signaling, and mechanical signals.

Wilding, J. P. H., Batterham, R. L., Davies, M., Van Gaal, L. F., Kandler, K., Konakli, K., Lingvay, I., McGowan, B. M., Oral, T. K., Rosenstock, J., Wadden, T. A., Wharton, S., Yokote, K., Zeuthen, N., Kushner, R. F., & STEP 1 Study Group. (2021). Once-weekly semaglutide in adults with overweight or obesity. *New England Journal of Medicine, 384*, 989–1002.

Re: Semaglutide 2.4 mg for obesity; STEP 1 weight-loss outcomes and DXA substudy context.

Wilding, J. P. H., Batterham, R. L., Calanna, S., Davies, M., Van Gaal, L. F., Lingvay, I., McGowan, B. M., Rosenstock, J., Tran, M. T. D., Wadden, T. A., Wharton, S., Yokote, K., Zeuthen, N., & Kushner, R. F. (2021). Impact of semaglutide on body composition in adults with overweight or obesity: Exploratory analysis of the STEP 1 study. *Journal of the Endocrine Society, 5*(Suppl. 1), A16–A17.

Re: Semaglutide body composition findings; fat mass reduction, lean mass reduction, and increased lean mass proportion.

Chapter 5

Dantzer, R., O'Connor, J. C., Freund, G. G., Johnson, R. W., & Kelley, K. W. (2008). From inflammation to sickness and depression: When the immune system subjugates the brain. *Nature Reviews Neuroscience, 9*(1), 46–56.

Re: Sickness behavior, fatigue, appetite suppression, social withdrawal, and brain–immune signaling during inflammatory states.

Dinarello, C. A. (2011). Interleukin-1 in the pathogenesis and treatment of inflammatory diseases. *Blood, 117*(14), 3720–3732.

Re: IL-1β biology, inflammatory activation, fever, and upstream cytokine signaling.

Ellingsgaard, H., Hauselmann, I., Schuler, B., Habib, A. M., Baggio, L. L., Meier, D. T., Eppler, E., Bouzakri, K., Wueest, S., Muller, Y. D., Hansen, A. M. K., Reinecke, M., Konrad, D., Gassmann, M., Reimann, F., Halban, P. A., Gromada, J., Drucker, D. J., Gribble, F. M., Ehses, J. A., & Donath, M. Y. (2011). Interleukin-6 enhances insulin secretion by increasing glucagon-like peptide-1 secretion from L cells and α cells. *Nature Medicine, 17*(11), 1481–1489.

Re: IL-6 stimulation of GLP-1 production from intestinal L cells and pancreatic alpha cells; immune–metabolic crosstalk.

Gutierrez, A. D., Gao, Z., Hamidi, V., Zhu, L., Saint Andre, K. B., Riggs, K., Ruscheinsky, M., Wang, H., Yu, Y., Miller, C., III, Vasquez, H., Taegtmeyer, H., & Kolonin, M. G. (2022). Anti-diabetic effects of GLP1 analogs are mediated by thermogenic interleukin-6 signaling in adipocytes. *Cell Reports Medicine, 3*(11), 100813.

Re: GLP-1 analogs, transient IL-6 upregulation, adipose IL-6 receptor signaling, thermogenic adipocyte browning, and STAT3 activation.

Hotamisligil, G. S. (2017). Inflammation, metaflammation and immunometabolic disorders. *Nature, 542*, 177–185.

Re: Immunometabolism, chronic low-grade inflammation, metabolic disease, and the limits of simplistic "inflammation is bad" framing.

Jones, B. E., Maerz, M. D., & Buckner, J. H. (2018). IL-6: A cytokine at the crossroads of autoimmunity. *Journal of Autoimmunity, 95*, 1–7.

Re: IL-6 signaling complexity, including classic signaling, trans-signaling, and cluster signaling/trans-presentation.

Kahles, F., Meyer, C., Möllmann, J., Diebold, S., Findeisen, H. M., Lebherz, C., Trautwein, C., Koch, A., Tacke, F., Marx, N., & Lehrke, M. (2014). GLP-1 secretion is increased by inflammatory stimuli in an IL-6–dependent manner, leading to hyperinsulinemia and blood glucose lowering. *Diabetes, 63*(10), 3221–3229.

Re: Inflammatory stimuli, IL-6–dependent GLP-1 secretion, and glucose-lowering responses.

Kang, S., Tanaka, T., Narazaki, M., & Kishimoto, T. (2019). Targeting interleukin-6 signaling in clinic. *Immunity, 50*(4), 1007–1023.

Re: IL-6 biology, classic and trans-signaling, inflammatory disease, and therapeutic targeting.

Kistner, T. M., Pedersen, B. K., & Lieberman, D. E. (2022). Interleukin 6 as an energy allocator in muscle tissue. *Nature Metabolism, 4*, 170–179.

Re: IL-6 as an energy allocation signal rather than a simple inflammatory marker.

Lebherz, C., Kahles, F., Piotrowski, K., Vogeser, M., Foldenauer, A. C., Nassau, K., Kilger, E., Marx, N., & Lehrke, M. (2016). Interleukin-6 predicts inflammation-induced increase of glucagon-like peptide-1 in humans in response to cardiac surgery with association to parameters of glucose metabolism. *Cardiovascular Diabetology, 15*, 21.

Re: Human evidence linking inflammation, IL-6, GLP-1 increases, and glucose metabolism during surgical inflammatory stress.

Londhe, P., & Guttridge, D. C. (2015). Inflammation induced loss of skeletal muscle. *Bone, 80*, 131–142.

Re: Inflammation, cytokines, cachexia, and loss of skeletal muscle.

Rose-John, S. (2023). Targeting IL-6 trans-signalling: Past, present and future prospects. *Nature Reviews Immunology, 23*, 666–681.

Re: IL-6 trans-signaling, soluble IL-6 receptor biology, and why total IL-6 values do not reveal pathway-specific activity.

Tsoli, M., & Robertson, G. (2013). Cancer cachexia: Malignant inflammation, tumorkines, and metabolic mayhem. *Trends in Endocrinology & Metabolism, 24*(4), 174–183.

Re: Cachexia as an inflammatory and metabolic wasting state involving altered energy use and tissue loss.

Wong, C. K., Drucker, D. J., & Baggio, L. L. (2025). Antiinflammatory actions of glucagon-like peptide-1–based therapies beyond metabolic benefits. *Journal of Clinical Investigation, 135*(18), e194751.

Re: GLP-1 medicines and anti-inflammatory actions across tissues; distinctions between metabolic, neural, immune, and non-immune mechanisms. This review also cautions that GLP-1 medicines modulate inflammation through multiple mechanisms, not a single uniform pathway.

Chapter 6

Baggio, L. L., & Drucker, D. J. (2014). Glucagon-like peptide-1 receptors in the brain: Controlling food intake and body weight. *Journal of Clinical Investigation, 124*(10), 4223–4226.

Re: Central GLP-1 receptor signaling, appetite regulation, and brain pathways relevant to long-term metabolic therapy.

Dantzer, R., O'Connor, J. C., Freund, G. G., Johnson, R. W., & Kelley, K. W. (2008). From inflammation to sickness and depression: When the immune system subjugates the brain. *Nature Reviews Neuroscience, 9*(1), 46–56.

Re: Cytokines, sickness behavior, appetite suppression, fatigue, mood changes, and brain–immune signaling.

Fischer, C. P. (2006). Interleukin-6 in acute exercise and training: What is the biological relevance? *Exercise Immunology Review, 12*, 6–33.

Re: Exercise-induced IL-6, transient cytokine pulses, substrate mobilization, and training adaptation.

Forcina, L., Miano, C., Pelosi, L., & Musarò, A. (2019). Signals from the niche: Insights into the role of IGF-1 and IL-6 in modulating skeletal muscle fibrosis. *Cells, 8*(3), 232.

Re: IL-6 in skeletal muscle repair, satellite-cell activity, fibrosis, and the difference between adaptive and maladaptive cytokine signaling.

Hathaway, J. T., Shah, M. P., Hathaway, D. B., Stewart, J. M., & Reddy, A. K. (2024). Risk of nonarteritic anterior ischemic optic neuropathy in patients prescribed semaglutide. *JAMA Ophthalmology, 142*(8), 732–739.

Re: Observational association between semaglutide prescription and NAION; hypothesis-generating rather than proof of causality. This was a matched cohort study and the authors emphasized the need for future study.

Hunter, C. A., & Jones, S. A. (2015). IL-6 as a keystone cytokine in health and disease. *Nature Immunology, 16*, 448–457.

Re: IL-6 as a pleiotropic cytokine with context-dependent roles in immunity, inflammation, tissue response, and disease.

Kistner, T. M., Pedersen, B. K., & Lieberman, D. E. (2022). Interleukin 6 as an energy allocator in muscle tissue. *Nature Metabolism, 4*, 170–179.

Re: IL-6 as an energy allocation signal, especially in skeletal muscle and exercise physiology.

Paolicelli, R. C., & Ferretti, M. T. (2017). Function and dysfunction of microglia during brain development: Consequences for synapses and neural circuits. *Frontiers in Synaptic Neuroscience, 9*, 9.

Re: Microglia, synaptic pruning, brain development, and consequences of altered neuroimmune signaling.

Pedersen, B. K., & Febbraio, M. A. (2008). Muscle as an endocrine organ: Focus on muscle-derived interleukin-6. *Physiological Reviews, 88*(4), 1379–1406.

Re: Muscle-derived IL-6, exercise, glucose mobilization, lipolysis, insulin sensitivity, and anti-inflammatory signaling.

Rose-John, S. (2023). Targeting IL-6 trans-signalling: Past, present and future prospects. *Nature Reviews Immunology, 23*, 666–681.

Re: IL-6 classic signaling, trans-signaling, soluble IL-6 receptor biology, and why total circulating IL-6 is not enough to infer function.

Schalbetter, S. M., von Arx, A. S., Cruz-Ochoa, N., Dawson, K., Ivanov, A., Mueller, F. S., Lin, H. Y., Amport, R., Beule, D., Zhang, P., et al. (2022). Adolescence is a sensitive period for prefrontal microglia to act on cognitive development. *Science Advances, 8*(9), eabi6672.

Re: Adolescence as a sensitive period for microglial effects on prefrontal cortex development and adult cognitive outcomes.

Stebegg, M., Kumar, S. D., Silva-Cayetano, A., Fonseca, V. R., Linterman, M. A., & Graca, L. (2018). Regulation of the germinal center response. *Frontiers in Immunology, 9*, 2469.

Re: Germinal-center biology, T follicular helper cells, B-cell maturation, antibody refinement, and cytokine regulation including IL-6.

Weghuber, D., Barrett, T., Barrientos-Pérez, M., Gies, I., Hesse, D., Jeppesen, O. K., Kelly, A. S., Mastrandrea, L. D., Sørrig, R., Arslanian, S., & STEP TEENS Investigators. (2022). Once-weekly semaglutide in adolescents with obesity. *New England Journal of Medicine, 387*, 2245–2257.

Re: Semaglutide in adolescents with obesity; efficacy and short-term safety, but not multi-decade developmental outcomes.

Wong, C. K., Drucker, D. J., & Baggio, L. L. (2025). Antiinflammatory actions of glucagon-like peptide-1–based therapies beyond metabolic benefits. *Journal of Clinical Investigation, 135*(18), e194751.

Re: GLP-1 medicines and anti-inflammatory actions across tissues; why "anti-inflammatory" is mechanistically more complicated than lowering CRP or IL-6 alone.

Chapter 7

Dulloo, A. G., Jacquet, J., Montani, J. P., & Schutz, Y. (2015). How dieting makes some fatter: From a perspective of human body composition autoregulation. *Proceedings of the Nutrition Society, 74*(4), 379–389.

Re: Body-composition autoregulation, fat regain, lean-mass deficits, and why repeated weight-loss/regain cycles can shift body composition.

Dulloo, A. G., Jacquet, J., Miles-Chan, J. L., & Schutz, Y. (2018). Collateral fattening in body composition autoregulation: Its determinants and significance for obesity predisposition. *European Journal of Clinical Nutrition, 72*, 657–664.

Re: Preferential fat regain, lean-mass lag, and the asymmetry between fat and lean tissue recovery after weight loss.

Fothergill, E., Guo, J., Howard, L., Kerns, J. C., Knuth, N. D., Brychta, R., Chen, K. Y., Skarulis, M. C., Walter, M., Walter, P. J., & Hall, K. D. (2016). Persistent metabolic adaptation 6 years after "The Biggest Loser" competition. *Obesity, 24*(8), 1612–1619.

Re: Persistent metabolic adaptation, reduced resting metabolic rate beyond that predicted by body composition, and long-term energy expenditure changes after major weight loss.

Hall, K. D., & Kahan, S. (2018). Maintenance of lost weight and long-term management of obesity. *Medical Clinics of North America, 102*(1), 183–197.

Re: Weight-loss maintenance, metabolic adaptation, appetite changes, behavioral pressure, and long-term obesity management.

Heymsfield, S. B., Gonzalez, M. C., Shen, W., Redman, L., & Thomas, D. (2014). Weight loss composition is one-fourth fat-free mass: A critical review and critique of this widely cited rule. *Obesity Reviews, 15*(4), 310–321.

Re: Composition of weight loss, variability in fat-free mass loss, and limitations of simple "rules" about lean mass loss.

Leibel, R. L., Rosenbaum, M., & Hirsch, J. (1995). Changes in energy expenditure resulting from altered body weight. *New England Journal of Medicine, 332*(10), 621–628.

Re: Reduced energy expenditure after weight loss and the biological defense of body weight.

MacLean, P. S., Bergouignan, A., Cornier, M. A., & Jackman, M. R. (2011). Biology's response to dieting: The impetus for weight regain. *American Journal of Physiology-Regulatory, Integrative and Comparative Physiology, 301*(3), R581–R600.

Re: Biological drivers of weight regain, including appetite, energy expenditure, fuel partitioning, and adaptive responses after dieting.

Rosenbaum, M., & Leibel, R. L. (2010). Adaptive thermogenesis in humans. *International Journal of Obesity, 34*(Suppl. 1), S47–S55.

Re: Adaptive thermogenesis, weight-reduced physiology, and persistent energy expenditure adaptation.

Spalding, K. L., Arner, E., Westermark, P. O., Bernard, S., Buchholz, B. A., Bergmann, O., Blomqvist, L., Hoffstedt, J., Näslund, E., Britton, T., Concha, H., Hassan, M., Rydén, M., Frisén, J., & Arner, P. (2008). Dynamics of fat cell turnover in humans. *Nature, 453*, 783–787.

Re: Adipocyte number, fat-cell turnover, and the finding that adipocyte number remains relatively stable in adulthood and after major weight loss.

Sumithran, P., Prendergast, L. A., Delbridge, E., Purcell, K., Shulkes, A., Kriketos, A., & Proietto, J. (2011). Long-term persistence of hormonal adaptations to weight loss. *New England Journal of Medicine, 365*, 1597–1604.

Re: Persistent appetite-hormone changes after weight loss, including signals favoring hunger and weight regain.

West, S., Scragg, J., Aveyard, P., Oke, J. L., Willis, L., & others. (2026). Weight regain after cessation of medication for weight management: Systematic review and meta-analysis. *BMJ, 392*, e085304.

Re: Weight regain after stopping weight-management medications, including GLP-1–based therapies; reversal of cardiometabolic improvements after cessation.

Wilding, J. P. H., Batterham, R. L., Davies, M., Van Gaal, L. F., Kandler, K., Konakli, K., Lingvay, I., McGowan, B. M., Oral, T. K., Rosenstock, J., Wadden, T. A., Wharton, S., Yokote, K., Zeuthen, N., & Kushner, R. F. (2022). Weight regain and cardiometabolic effects after withdrawal of semaglutide: The STEP 1 trial extension. *Diabetes, Obesity and Metabolism, 24*(8), 1553–1564.

Re: Weight regain and reversal of cardiometabolic improvements one year after semaglutide withdrawal.

Chapter 8

Apovian, C. M., Aronne, L. J., Bessesen, D. H., McDonnell, M. E., Murad, M. H., Pagotto, U., Ryan, D. H., Still, C. D., & Endocrine Society. (2015). Pharmacological management of obesity: An Endocrine Society clinical practice guideline. *Journal of Clinical Endocrinology & Metabolism, 100*(2), 342–362.

Re: Obesity pharmacotherapy, medication selection, risk–benefit evaluation, and long-term clinical management.

Berning, P., Srivastava, G., Uzoigwe, C., & colleagues. (2025). Longitudinal analysis of obesity drug use and public interest in the United States. *JAMA Network Open, 8*(1), e2457062.

Re: U.S. obesity medication prescribing trends, public interest, and phentermine prescription volume over time.

Bray, G. A., Ryan, D. H., & Wilding, J. P. H. (2023). Pharmacologic treatment of obesity. *New England Journal of Medicine, 389*, 2565–2578.

Re: Modern obesity pharmacotherapy, including sympathomimetic agents, GLP-1 receptor agonists, dual agonists, efficacy, safety, and long-term treatment framing.

Gasoyan, H., Pfoh, E. R., Schauer, P. R., Rothberg, M. B., & colleagues. (2025). Changes in weight and glycemic control following obesity treatment with semaglutide or tirzepatide by discontinuation status. *Obesity*.

Re: Real-world semaglutide/tirzepatide outcomes; lower weight loss than clinical trials, high use of lower maintenance doses, and reduced efficacy with discontinuation. In this Cleveland Clinic cohort of 7,881 patients, 80.8% had low maintenance dosages and mean one-year weight reduction was 8.7% overall.

Hendricks, E. J., Greenway, F. L., Westman, E. C., & Gupta, A. K. (2011). Blood pressure and heart rate effects, weight loss and maintenance during long-term phentermine pharmacotherapy for obesity. *Obesity, 19*(12), 2351–2360.

Re: Long-term observational phentermine use, weight loss, blood pressure, and heart-rate effects in clinical practice.

Hendricks, E. J., Srisurapanont, M., Schmidt, S. L., & Greenway, F. L. (2014). Addiction potential of phentermine prescribed during long-term treatment of obesity. *International Journal of Obesity, 38*(2), 292–298.

Re: Phentermine abuse/dependence concerns and long-term clinical use.

Lewis, K. H., Fischer, H., Ard, J., Barton, L., Bessesen, D. H., Daley, M. F., Desai, J., Horberg, M. A., Koebnick, C., Oshiro, C. E., Yamamoto, A., Young, D. R., & Tajeu, G. S. (2019). Safety and effectiveness of longer-term phentermine use: Clinical outcomes from an electronic health record cohort. *Obesity, 27*(4), 591–602.

Re: Longer-term phentermine use, weight loss, and cardiovascular safety outcomes in a large EHR cohort.

Novo Nordisk. (2025). *Wegovy® (semaglutide) prescribing information*. U.S. Food and Drug Administration.

Re: Semaglutide dosing, dose escalation, adverse effects, pharmacokinetics, half-life, and obesity indication.

Rubino, D., Abrahamsson, N., Davies, M., Hesse, D., Greenway, F. L., Jensen, C., Lingvay, I., Mosenzon, O., Rosenstock, J., Rubio, M. A., Rudofsky, G., Tadayon, S., Wadden, T. A., Dicker, D., & STEP 4 Investigators. (2021). Effect of continued weekly subcutaneous semaglutide vs placebo on weight loss maintenance in adults with overweight or obesity: The STEP 4 randomized clinical trial. *JAMA, 325*(14), 1414–1425.

Re: Semaglutide continuation versus withdrawal; ongoing treatment maintained weight loss, while withdrawal led to regain.

U.S. Drug Enforcement Administration. (2024). *Controlled substances: Alphabetical order*. Diversion Control Division.

Re: Federal controlled-substance scheduling; phentermine as Schedule IV and amphetamine products as Schedule II.

U.S. Food and Drug Administration. (2012). *Adipex-P® (phentermine hydrochloride) prescribing information.*

Re: Phentermine indication for short-term obesity treatment, dosing, contraindications, warnings, and adverse reactions. The FDA label describes phentermine as a short-term adjunct to exercise, behavioral modification, and caloric restriction.

U.S. Food and Drug Administration. (2025). *Adderall XR® (mixed salts of a single-entity amphetamine product) prescribing information.*

Re: ADHD stimulant labeling, Schedule II status, blood pressure and heart-rate effects, abuse potential, and monitoring.

U.S. Food and Drug Administration. (2026). *Zepbound® (tirzepatide) prescribing information.*

Re: Tirzepatide dosing, dose escalation, adverse effects, pharmacokinetics, half-life, and chronic weight-management indication.

Wilding, J. P. H., Batterham, R. L., Calanna, S., Davies, M., Van Gaal, L. F., Lingvay, I., McGowan, B. M., Rosenstock, J., Tran, M. T. D., Wadden, T. A., Wharton, S., Yokote, K., Zeuthen, N., Kushner, R. F., & STEP 1 Study Group. (2021). Once-weekly semaglutide in adults with overweight or obesity. *New England Journal of Medicine, 384*, 989–1002.

Re: STEP 1 semaglutide obesity trial; 14.9% mean weight loss at 68 weeks and gastrointestinal adverse-event discontinuation.

Wilding, J. P. H., Batterham, R. L., Davies, M., Van Gaal, L. F., Kandler, K., Konakli, K., Lingvay, I., McGowan, B. M., Oral, T. K., Rosenstock, J., Wadden, T. A., Wharton, S., Yokote, K., Zeuthen, N., & Kushner, R. F. (2022). Weight regain and cardiometabolic effects after withdrawal of semaglutide: The STEP 1 trial extension. *Diabetes, Obesity and Metabolism, 24*(8), 1553–1564.

Re: Weight regain after semaglutide withdrawal and reversal of cardiometabolic improvements.

Chapter 9

Atherton, P. J., & Smith, K. (2012). Muscle protein synthesis in response to nutrition and exercise. *Journal of Physiology, 590*(5), 1049–1057.

Re: Muscle protein synthesis, amino-acid signaling, and the interaction between protein nutrition and exercise.

Cava, E., Yeat, N. C., & Mittendorfer, B. (2017). Preserving healthy muscle during weight loss. *Advances in Nutrition, 8*(3), 511–519.

Re: Lean mass loss during weight reduction and the roles of protein intake, resistance training, and energy balance in muscle preservation.

Heymsfield, S. B., Gonzalez, M. C., Shen, W., Redman, L., & Thomas, D. (2014). Weight loss composition is one-fourth fat-free mass: A critical review and critique of this widely cited rule. *Obesity Reviews, 15*(4), 310–321.

Re: Variability in lean mass/fat-free mass loss during weight reduction and why simple rules require clinical context.

International Agency for Research on Cancer. (2024). *IARC Handbooks of Cancer Prevention Volume 20A: Reduction or cessation of alcohol consumption.* International Agency for Research on Cancer.

Re: Alcoholic beverages as Group 1 carcinogens and cancer-risk rationale for advising avoidance. IARC notes that alcoholic beverages were first classified as carcinogenic to humans in 1987, with later additions of colorectal and female breast cancer to the list of alcohol-caused cancers.

Layman, D. K., Anthony, T. G., Rasmussen, B. B., Adams, S. H., Lynch, C. J., Brinkworth, G. D., & Davis, T. A. (2015). Defining meal requirements for protein to optimize metabolic roles of amino acids. *American Journal of Clinical Nutrition, 101*(6), 1330S–1338S.

Re: Per-meal protein thresholds, leucine signaling, and the clinical practicality of distributing meaningful protein doses across meals.

Layman, D. K., Hudson, J. L., Erickson, D. J., & Baum, J. I. (2024). Impacts of protein quantity and distribution on body composition, muscle function, and health outcomes in adults. *Frontiers in Nutrition, 11*, 1388986.

Re: Protein quantity, protein distribution, leucine thresholds, meal-based protein dosing, body composition, and muscle function.

Loenneke, J. P., Loprinzi, P. D., Murphy, C. H., & Phillips, S. M. (2016). Per meal dose and frequency of protein consumption is associated with lean mass and muscle performance. *Clinical Nutrition, 35*(6), 1506–1511.

Re: Associations between per-meal protein intake, lean mass, and muscle performance; supports practical meal-based protein framing.

Lopez, P., Taaffe, D. R., Galvão, D. A., Newton, R. U., Nonemacher, E. R., Wendt, V. M., & Pinto, R. S. (2022). Resistance training effectiveness on body composition and body weight outcomes in individuals with overweight and obesity across the lifespan: A systematic review and meta-analysis. *Obesity Reviews, 23*(5), e13428.

Re: Resistance training as a key strategy for preserving or improving lean tissue and strength during obesity treatment.

Parr, E. B., Camera, D. M., Areta, J. L., Burke, L. M., Phillips, S. M., Hawley, J. A., & Coffey, V. G. (2014). Alcohol ingestion impairs maximal post-exercise rates of myofibrillar protein synthesis following a single bout of concurrent training. *PLOS ONE, 9*(2), e88384.

Re: Alcohol suppressing post-exercise muscle protein synthesis, even when co-ingested with protein, and the relevance of alcohol avoidance for muscle recovery.

Phillips, S. M. (2016). The impact of protein quality on the promotion of resistance exercise-induced changes in muscle mass. *Nutrition & Metabolism, 13*, 64.

Re: Protein quality, amino-acid composition, resistance exercise, and muscle adaptation.

Ponti, F., Santoro, A., Mercatelli, D., Gasperini, C., Conte, M., Martucci, M., Sangiorgi, L., Franceschi, C., & Bazzocchi, A. (2019). Aging and imaging assessment of body composition: From fat to facts. *Frontiers in Endocrinology, 10*, 861.

Re: DXA/body composition assessment, fat mass, lean mass, bone parameters, and clinical interpretation during aging and weight change.

Rubino, D., Abrahamsson, N., Davies, M., Hesse, D., Greenway, F. L., Jensen, C., Lingvay, I., Mosenzon, O., Rosenstock, J., Rubio, M. A., Rudofsky, G., Tadayon, S., Wadden, T. A., Dicker, D., & STEP 4 Investigators. (2021). Effect of continued weekly subcutaneous semaglutide vs placebo on weight loss maintenance in adults with overweight or obesity: The STEP 4 randomized clinical trial. *JAMA, 325*(14), 1414–1425.

Re: Continued semaglutide treatment versus withdrawal and the role of ongoing pharmacotherapy in weight-loss maintenance.

Schoenfeld, B. J., & Aragon, A. A. (2018). How much protein can the body use in a single meal for muscle-building? Implications for daily protein distribution. *Journal of the International Society of Sports Nutrition, 15*, 10.

Re: Per-meal protein dose, muscle protein synthesis, and practical implications for protein distribution across the day.

Wilding, J. P. H., Batterham, R. L., Calanna, S., Davies, M., Van Gaal, L. F., Lingvay, I., McGowan, B. M., Rosenstock, J., Tran, M. T. D., Wadden, T. A., Wharton, S., Yokote, K., Zeuthen, N., Kushner, R. F., & STEP 1 Study Group. (2021). Once-weekly semaglutide in adults with overweight or obesity. *New England Journal of Medicine, 384*, 989–1002.

Re: Semaglutide 2.4 mg obesity trial, weight loss efficacy, adverse events, and DXA substudy showing greater fat mass than lean mass reduction.

Wilding, J. P. H., Batterham, R. L., Davies, M., Van Gaal, L. F., Kandler, K., Konakli, K., Lingvay, I., McGowan, B. M., Oral, T. K., Rosenstock, J., Wadden, T. A., Wharton, S., Yokote, K., Zeuthen, N., & Kushner, R. F. (2022). Weight regain and cardiometabolic effects after withdrawal of semaglutide: The STEP 1 trial extension. *Diabetes, Obesity and Metabolism, 24*(8), 1553–1564.

Re: Weight regain after semaglutide withdrawal; participants regained about two-thirds of prior weight loss one year after stopping therapy.

Chapter 10

Alhadeff, A. L., Rupprecht, L. E., & Hayes, M. R. (2012). GLP-1 neurons in the nucleus of the solitary tract project directly to the ventral tegmental area and nucleus accumbens to control for food intake. *Endocrinology, 153*(2), 647–658.

Re: Central GLP-1 neurons, reward circuitry, food intake, and the neural axis connecting satiety with motivation.

Anker, S. D., Morley, J. E., & von Haehling, S. (2016). Welcome to the ICD-10 code for sarcopenia. *Journal of Cachexia, Sarcopenia and Muscle, 7*(5), 512–514.

Re: Sarcopenia as a clinically recognized condition and the importance of muscle loss as more than a cosmetic or body-composition detail.

Brodney, S., Valentine, K. D., Sepucha, K., Fowler, F. J., & Barry, M. J. (2021). Patient preference distribution for use of statin therapy. *JAMA Network Open, 4*(3), e210661.

Re: Patient preferences for statin therapy after absolute benefit and harm information; supports broader shared decision-making rather than automatic guideline application. In this study, only 45.1% of participants would definitely or probably choose statin therapy after reviewing personalized benefit/harm information, and 75% preference was not reached until a 20% 10-year risk threshold.

Cava, E., Yeat, N. C., & Mittendorfer, B. (2017). Preserving healthy muscle during weight loss. *Advances in Nutrition, 8*(3), 511–519.

Re: Lean mass loss during weight reduction and the role of protein, resistance training, and energy balance in muscle preservation.

Clemmensen, C., Müller, T. D., Woods, S. C., Berthoud, H. R., Seeley, R. J., & Tschöp, M. H. (2017). Gut-brain cross-talk in metabolic control. *Cell, 168*(5), 758–774.

Re: Gut–brain signaling, appetite regulation, metabolic control, and why GLP-1 biology cannot be reduced to a single peripheral hormone effect.

Cruz-Jentoft, A. J., & Sayer, A. A. (2019). Sarcopenia. *The Lancet, 393*(10191), 2636–2646.

Re: Sarcopenia definitions, muscle strength/function, aging, mortality, and clinical consequences.

Dulloo, A. G., Jacquet, J., Miles-Chan, J. L., & Schutz, Y. (2018). Collateral fattening in body composition autoregulation: Its determinants and significance for obesity predisposition. *European Journal of Clinical Nutrition, 72*, 657–664.

Re: Fat regain, lean-mass deficits, and why repeated weight loss/regain can worsen body composition over time.

Fried, L. P., Tangen, C. M., Walston, J., Newman, A. B., Hirsch, C., Gottdiener, J., Seeman, T., Tracy, R., Kop, W. J., Burke, G., & McBurnie, M. A. (2001). Frailty in older adults: Evidence for a phenotype. *Journals of Gerontology: Series A, 56*(3), M146–M156.

Re: Frailty phenotype: weight loss, weakness, exhaustion, slow gait speed, and low physical activity.

Gerstein, H. C., Colhoun, H. M., Dagenais, G. R., Diaz, R., Lakshmanan, M., Pais, P., Probstfield, J., Riesmeyer, J. S., Riddle, M. C., Rydén, L., Xavier, D., Atisso, C. M., Dyal, L., Hall, S., Rao-Melacini, P., Wong, G., Avezum, A., Basile, J., Chung, N., Conget, I., Cushman, W. C., Franek, E., Hancu, N., Hanefeld, M., Holt, S., Jansky, P., Keltai, M., Lanas, F., Leiter, L. A., Lopez-Jaramillo, P., Lytvyn, L., Mazzone, T., Meaney, E., Nesto, R., Pan, C.,

Pratley, R. E., & Ramasundarahettige, C. (2019). Dulaglutide and cardiovascular outcomes in type 2 diabetes (REWIND): A double-blind, randomised placebo-controlled trial. *The Lancet, 394*(10193), 121–130.

Re: REWIND trial; dulaglutide, MACE reduction, broader T2D population, lower baseline risk, and smaller absolute benefit.

Heymsfield, S. B., Gonzalez, M. C., Shen, W., Redman, L., & Thomas, D. (2014). Weight loss composition is one-fourth fat-free mass: A critical review and critique of this widely cited rule. *Obesity Reviews, 15*(4), 310–321.

Re: Composition of weight loss, variability in fat-free mass loss, and limits of simple lean-mass rules.

Jastreboff, A. M., Kaplan, L. M., Frías, J. P., Wu, Q., Du, Y., Gurbuz, S., Coskun, T., Haupt, A., Milicevic, Z., Hartman, M. L., & Retatrutide Phase 2 Obesity Trial Investigators. (2023). Triple–hormone-receptor agonist retatrutide for obesity. *New England Journal of Medicine, 389*, 514–526.

Re: Triple agonism, major weight loss, and the expanding potency of endocrine-combination obesity pharmacotherapy.

Kongnakorn, T., Migliaccio-Walle, K., Jiao, T., Caro, J. J., & Getsios, D. (2009). Economic evaluation of atorvastatin for prevention of cardiovascular events in patients with hypertension and additional risk factors. *Value in Health, 12*(1), 65–72.

Re: ASCOT-LLA modeling; estimated mean lifetime gains in life-years and QALYs per treated patient.

Layman, D. K., Anthony, T. G., Rasmussen, B. B., Adams, S. H., Lynch, C. J., Brinkworth, G. D., & Davis, T. A. (2015). Defining meal requirements for protein to optimize metabolic roles of amino acids. *American Journal of Clinical Nutrition, 101*(6), 1330S–1338S.

Re: Per-meal protein thresholds, leucine signaling, and practical protein-distribution logic relevant to muscle preservation.

Luo, Y., Kawakami, H., Funada, S., et al. (2026). Measuring public preferences for statin therapy using the smallest worthwhile difference. *JAMA Internal Medicine, 186*(4), 488–490.

Re: Public preference thresholds for statin therapy; many respondents wanted larger absolute benefits than standard statin trials usually provide before considering treatment worthwhile.

Marso, S. P., Daniels, G. H., Brown-Frandsen, K., Kristensen, P., Mann, J. F. E., Nauck, M. A., Nissen, S. E., Pocock, S., Poulter, N. R., Ravn, L. S., Steinberg, W. M., Stockner, M., Zinman, B., Bergenstal, R. M., Buse, J. B., & LEADER Steering Committee. (2016). Liraglutide and cardiovascular outcomes in type 2 diabetes. *New England Journal of Medicine, 375*, 311–322.

Re: LEADER trial; liraglutide cardiovascular outcomes, high-risk T2D population, MACE reduction, and absolute benefit.

Marso, S. P., Bain, S. C., Consoli, A., Eliaschewitz, F. G., Jódar, E., Leiter, L. A., Lingvay, I., Rosenstock, J., Seufert, J., Warren, M. L., Woo, V., Hansen, O., Holst, A. G., Pettersson, J., Vilsbøll, T., & SUSTAIN-6 Investigators. (2016). Semaglutide and cardiovascular outcomes in patients with type 2 diabetes. *New England Journal of Medicine, 375*, 1834–1844.

Re: SUSTAIN-6 trial; semaglutide cardiovascular safety and MACE reduction in high-risk T2D.

Nauck, M. A., & Meier, J. J. (2021). The incretin effect in healthy individuals and those with type 2 diabetes: Physiology, pathophysiology, and response to therapeutic interventions. *The Lancet Diabetes & Endocrinology, 9*(10), 689–704.

Re: Incretin physiology, GLP-1/GIP biology, type 2 diabetes, and therapeutic incretin responses.

Redfern, J., et al. (2026). Effectiveness of data-driven quality improvement on hospitalizations and health outcomes for people with coronary heart disease in primary care (QUEL): A cluster randomized controlled trial with 24-month follow-up. *Circulation: Cardiovascular Quality and Outcomes.*

Re: Data-driven collaborative quality improvement in primary care for coronary heart disease; no significant improvement in unplanned cardiovascular hospitalizations, MACE, prescribing, risk-factor targets, or management planning at 24 months.

Rosenbaum, M., & Leibel, R. L. (2010). Adaptive thermogenesis in humans. *International Journal of Obesity, 34*(Suppl. 1), S47–S55.

Re: Weight-reduced physiology, adaptive thermogenesis, and why weight loss does not simply return the body to a prior metabolic state.

Sever, P. S., Dahlöf, B., Poulter, N. R., Wedel, H., Beevers, G., Caulfield, M., Collins, R., Kjeldsen, S. E., Kristinsson, A., McInnes, G. T., Mehlsen, J., Nieminen, M., O'Brien, E., & Östergren, J. (2003). Prevention of coronary and stroke events with atorvastatin in hypertensive patients who have average or lower-than-average cholesterol concentrations, in the Anglo-Scandinavian Cardiac Outcomes Trial—Lipid Lowering Arm (ASCOT-LLA): A multicentre randomised controlled trial. *The Lancet, 361*(9364), 1149–1158.

Re: ASCOT-LLA; statin primary prevention trial illustrating relative versus absolute risk interpretation.

Simpson, S. J., & Raubenheimer, D. (2005). Obesity: The protein leverage hypothesis. *Obesity Reviews, 6*(2), 133–142.

Re: Protein leverage hypothesis; protein dilution as a driver of excess energy intake.

Solon-Biet, S. M., McMahon, A. C., Ballard, J. W. O., Ruohonen, K., Wu, L. E., Cogger, V. C., Warren, A., Huang, X., Pichaud, N., Melvin, R. G., Gokarn, R., Khalil, M., Turner, N., Cooney, G. J., Sinclair, D. A., Raubenheimer, D., Le Couteur, D. G., & Simpson, S. J. (2014). The ratio of macronutrients, not caloric intake, dictates cardiometabolic health, aging, and longevity in ad libitum-fed mice. *Cell Metabolism, 19*(3), 418–430.

Re: Macronutrient ratio, protein dilution, hyperphagia, and appetite as nutrient-regulated rather than calorie-regulated alone.

Teff, K. L., Rickels, M. R., Grudziak, J., Fuller, C., Nguyen, H. L., & Rickels, M. R. (2010). Anticipatory hormonal responses to food intake. *Endocrinology and Metabolism Clinics of North America, 39*(2), 253–272.

Re: Anticipatory metabolic signaling and the broader point that appetite and nutrient handling are coordinated before and during intake.

van Bloemendaal, L., IJzerman, R. G., ten Kulve, J. S., Barkhof, F., Konrad, R. J., Drent, M. L., Veltman, D. J., Diamant, M., & la Fleur, S. E. (2014). GLP-1 receptor activation modulates appetite- and reward-related brain areas in humans. *Diabetes, 63*(12), 4186–4196.

Re: Human neuroimaging evidence that GLP-1 receptor activation alters appetite and reward-related brain responses.

Wilding, J. P. H., Batterham, R. L., Calanna, S., Davies, M., Van Gaal, L. F., Lingvay, I., McGowan, B. M., Rosenstock, J., Tran, M. T. D., Wadden, T. A., Wharton, S., Yokote, K., Zeuthen, N., Kushner, R. F., & STEP 1 Study Group. (2021). Once-weekly semaglutide in adults with overweight or obesity. *New England Journal of Medicine, 384*, 989–1002.

Re: STEP 1 semaglutide obesity trial; weight loss, adverse events, and DXA substudy showing fat and lean mass changes.

Author Bio

Vyvyane Loh, MD is a board-certified Internal Medicine and Obesity Medicine physician, writer, and educator. For more than two decades, she has worked at the intersection of metabolism, appetite, body composition, immune signaling, and the long arc of chronic disease.

A former Radcliffe Fellow and Guggenheim Fellow in Fiction, Dr. Loh brings a rare cross-disciplinary lens to medicine, combining scientific rigor with literary attention to structure, meaning, and human experience. Trained in medicine but drawn equally to language and systems, she writes at the edge of physiology and culture. She is interested not only in what the body does, but in how modern life reshapes the conditions for health.

Her work is marked by a systems-based approach to medicine and a commitment to making complex biological ideas intellectually rigorous, clinically grounded, and deeply readable. She is the founder of **Wellth-e**, an independent medical e-zine dedicated to clear, thoughtful science and medicine for readers who want more than headlines and generic health advice.

The Architecture of Enough reflects her ongoing interest in the places where medicine, biology, and human experience fail to line up neatly, and in the questions that begin there.

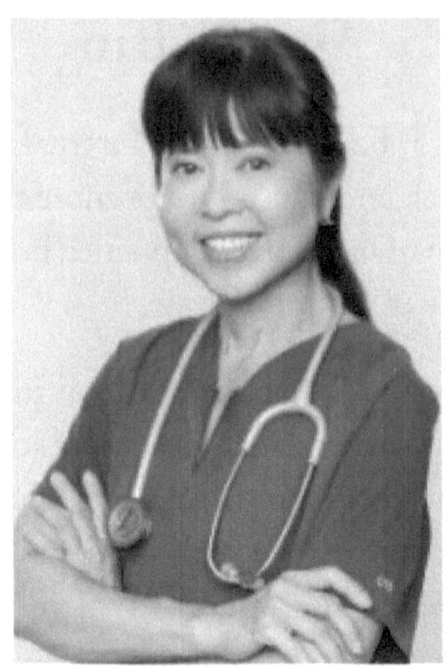

Find Dr. Loh

For Dr. Loh's writing, teaching, videos, newsletter, and future projects, visit vyvyanelohmd.com[1].

For speaking, interviews, or professional inquiries, contact vlmdpodcast@gmail.com.

1. http://vyvyanelohmd.com

Acknowledgements:

This book was shaped by more people than I can name here: patients, teachers, colleagues, readers, friends, and family members whose questions, trust, skepticism, and encouragement challenged me to think more clearly.

I am especially grateful to those who have allowed me to sit with them in the difficult spaces where biology, illness, uncertainty, and ordinary life meet. This book grew out of those conversations.

To everyone who has helped me keep asking better questions: thank you.

Continue the conversation

If this book opened your mind to the power of better questions, explore **Wellth-e** — my independent medical-science letter on metabolism, medicine, the body, and the systems that shape health.

Scan to read free issues and future essays at https://wellth-e.com/main-issues/

www.ingramcontent.com/pod-product-compliance
Lightning Source LLC
LaVergne TN
LVHW090514110826
845146LV00003B/851

* 9 7 9 8 9 9 5 4 9 7 9 1 2 *